Third Edition

Pediatric Hair Disorders
An Atlas and Text

Pediatric Diagnosis and Management
Series Editors: James F. Bale Jr. and Stephen D. Marks

NEW AND FORTHCOMING TITLES

Third Edition

Pediatric Hair Disorders
An Atlas and Text

Juan Ferrando, PhD, MD
Consultant in Dermatology
Hospital Clínic
and Associate Professor of Dermatology
Universitat de Barcelona, Spain

Ramon Grimalt, PhD, MD
Associate Professor of Dermatology
Faculty of Medicine and Health Sciences
Universitat Internacional de Catalunya
Barcelona, Spain

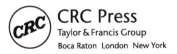

CRC Press
Taylor & Francis Group
Boca Raton London New York

CRC Press is an imprint of the
Taylor & Francis Group, an **informa** business

CRC Press
Taylor & Francis Group
6000 Broken Sound Parkway NW, Suite 300
Boca Raton, FL 33487-2742

© 2017 by Taylor & Francis Group, LLC
CRC Press is an imprint of Taylor & Francis Group, an Informa business

No claim to original U.S. Government works

Printed on acid-free paper
Version Date: 20160620

International Standard Book Number-13: 978-1-4987-0777-0 (Paperback)

Visit the Taylor & Francis Web site at
http://www.taylorandfrancis.com

and the CRC Press Web site at
http://www.crcpress.com

To my wife, Dra. Esperanza Navarra; to my sons and daughter, David,

Marc, and Anna; and to my granddaughter, Jana.

Juan Ferrando

To my wife, Dra. Alicia Mirada, and to my daughters, Rita and Gina.

Ramon Grimalt

Contents

Foreword

Hair diseases represent a significant portion of cases seen by pediatric dermatologists. It is, therefore, a great pleasure to see the publication of this diagnostic atlas for pediatric hair disorders. The authors are well known in international trichology, especially in the field of hair problems in childhood. This book is easy to follow and represents a timely contribution to both clinical dermatology and pediatrics.

During the past decade, many investigators involved in clinical and basic research have been attracted by the field of hair disorders. In particular, molecular analysis of genetic hair disorders is developing rapidly. The examination of the status of hair growth, including microscopic analysis of hair shafts, represents a visual approach that may yield important hints for the diagnosis of complex genetic syndromes. This book will help both dermatologists and pediatricians improve their skills in the differential diagnosis of hair diseases.

Why *pediatric* trichology? For many reasons it is necessary to treat the special problems of hair diseases of children. For example, the full-blown picture of Menkes' kinky hair disease is virtually never seen in adult patients. Loose anagen hair very rarely occurs in adults, and trichotillomania is far more frequently seen in childhood.

Dermatologists are in the enviable situation of being able to study many disorders with simple diagnostic techniques. Hair is easily accessible to examination but, paradoxically, hair examination is often ignored by non-dermatologists. The present text will serve as an important tool in the diagnostic processes used in daily practice, and it will help, for example, to distinguish certain acquired and genetically determined hair diseases. The informative iconographic material of this book will stimulate and encourage physicians to perform microscopic analyses of hair shafts and cooperate with dermatologists experienced in this special field of medicine.

It is a privilege to be associated, even in this peripheral form, with this text that will be a most welcome addition for all those dealing with hair diseases of children.

Rudolf Happle, M.D.
Marburg, Germany

Preface

Pediatric trichology covers a wide field of study that includes pediatric and dermatological cases. It comprises extremely common entities (alopecia areata, trichotillomania) and others that are rare and more difficult to diagnose (hair dysplasias, genodermatosis). In many of the clinical pictures, hair alteration (diffuse or localized, alopecia, cicatricial or non-cicatricial, acquired or congenital) is a fundamental clue for clinical diagnosis (Menkes syndrome, Netherton syndrome, trichothiodystrophy). Knowledge of the possible clinical associations in all these entities (follicular hyperkeratosis, ichthyosis, cataracts, seizures) may also contribute to a diagnosis.

The personal experience of one of us (JF) over the last 35 years with regard to many of these entities made it possible to present the clinical pictures herein with the basic idea of helping with the diagnoses of the various clinically described syndromes. This book is composed not only of the clinical pictures but also of key histopathological, microscopic, and scanning electron microscopy findings. In some cases, the findings of x-ray microanalysis (trichothiodystrophy, green hair) are pointed out. We believe that it is also important to emphasize other aspects that have interested us, such as the therapeutic approach to each entity and a basic bibliography pointing out our contributions and views on each subject and those of others. An extensive index and a glossary of terms are included to aid consultation.

Finally we would like to add that this book constitutes a new and revised version of the second edition of the *Atlas of Diagnosis in Pediatric Trichology*, after the first Spanish version published in 1996 (*Atlas de Diagnóstico en Tricología Pediátrica*, Aula Médica, Madrid). The warm welcome given to this first edition and healthy sales of the second encouraged us to go ahead with a new extended third version of the book.

Our sincere hope is that our *Pediatric Hair Disorders*, now in its third edition and full of clinical pictures followed by clear and concise text, will help you with the diagnosis of each entity. We would like this book to assist you in solving any doubts that hair diseases—especially in our smallest patients—may pose to you. Finally, we truly hope it will be useful to our dermatologist colleagues and also to pediatricians interested in trichology.

Juan Ferrando
Ramon Grimalt

Acknowledgments

We would like to thank Rudolf Happle for writing his kind Foreword and support of this project. We also thank the following contributors who helped by providing clinical pictures for the atlas: Ulrike Blume-Peytavi, Francisco Camacho, Stefano Cambiaghi, Koenrad Devriendt, Marie L. Geerts, G. G. Lestringant, and Pablo de Unamuno, as well as Ramon Fontarnau, Francisco Javier García Veigas, and Anna Domínguez of the Electron Microscopy Unit of the University of Barcelona for their years of collaboration on scanning electron microscopy and x-ray microanalysis research on hair.

Introduction

Trichology, as we all know, studies the normal condition of hair and the pilosebaceous unit along with the prevention and treatment of all their pathological processes. It does not usually take into account tumors of the pilosebaceous follicles, but rather deals primarily with inflammatory and toxic processes or conditions with other origins (e.g., systemic diseases).

In most cases, the pathologies lead to a common clinical sign: alopecia. Nevertheless, we must distinguish congenital hair loss (atrichia or hypotrichosis) from acquired hair loss or alopecia. Either of these forms of alopecia may be cicatricial or non-cicatricial, depending on whether permanent follicular damage is present or the damage is transitory and can be repaired.

In cicatricial alopecia, clinically irregular plaques with the persistence of some hair can be observed and cutaneous surfaces show alterations (erythema, follicular depressions, fibrosis). In non-cicatricial alopecia (for example, alopecia areata), the skin has a normal appearance and the plaques are rounded and well shaped. From a histological view, chronic follicular damage (atrophy, fibrosis, remains of chronic inflammatory infiltrate) is observed in cicatricial alopecia. In non-cicatricial alopecia (alopecia areata), inflammatory infiltrates can also be observed but there is no permanent damage to follicles. It is not possible to recover from cicatricial alopecia, whereas for non-cicatricial alopecia (alopecia areata, effluvium) full recovery (except for androgenic alopecia) can be achieved.

Other hair pathologies are not related primarily to alopecia but rather to alterations of the hair shaft (hair shaft dysplasia, external causes) or changes in color (graying and green hair).

We list below several general reference books on trichology—both classics and the most recent:

Camacho FM, Randall VA, and Price VH. *Hair and Its Disorders: Biology, Pathology, and Management*. London: Martin Dunitz, 2000.

Camacho FM, Tosti A, Randall VA, and Price VH. *Montagna Tricología*, 3rd ed. Madrid: Grupo Aula Médica, 2013.

Dawber R and Van Neste D. *Hair and Scalp Disorders*. London: Martin Dunitz, 1995.

Olsen EA. *Disorders of Hair Growth: Diagnosis and Treatment*, 2nd ed. New York: McGraw-Hill, 2003.

Rook A and Dawber R. *Diseases of the Hair and Scalp*. Oxford: Blackwell Scientific, 1991.

Shapiro J and Otberg N. *Hair Loss and Restoration*, 2nd ed. Boca Raton, FL: CRC Press, 2015.

Sinclair RD, Banfield CC, and Dawber RPR. *Handbook of Diseases of the Hair and Scalp*. Oxford: Blackwell Scientific, 1999.

Tosti A. *Dermoscopy of Hair and Nail Disorders*, 2nd ed. Boca Raton, FL: CRC Press, 2015.

1

Hair Shaft Dysplasias

Hair shaft dysplasias are malformations of hair shafts. Most cases are congenital, hereditary or not; others are acquired (e.g., bubble hair). The malformations may involve a localized or generalized defect, but always follow a characteristic morphologic pattern [1,2]. The defects may be restricted to the hair or even constitute a diagnostic clue pointing to a genodermatosis (e.g., Netherton syndrome, trichothiodystrophy). Classification of hair shaft dysplasias is difficult but for practical purposes we accept the scheme shown in Table 1.1 [2,3].

Monilethrix (Beaded Hair)

Monilethrix is an autosomal dominant (AD) defect of the hair shaft characterized by short hair, only a few millimeters long and beaded. Breaking of the hair shaft occurs as soon as hair emerges from the ostium folliculorum due to narrowing of the shaft segments. Focal follicular hyperkeratosis and marked hypotrichosis may also be seen. Monilethrix generally affects individuals of different generations of the same family. The morphological defect is the periodic narrowing of the hair shaft that may be seen deep in hair follicles in biopsy specimens [4,5].

Genetics: Monilethrix is an AD hereditary defect caused by mutation of genes *hHb1*, *hHb3*, and *hHb6* localized on chromosome (cr) 12q13 that encode diverse trichokeratins. We have recently reported a new family with a change in the nucleotide in heterozygosis at position 154 of exon1 of gene *KRT81* (154 G > C). In the DNA sequence, this substitution involves a change of one amino acid in a protein (glycine for arginine at position 52) [6]. Interruption of keratin synthesis may be the cause of periodic variations of hair shaft diameter. Autosomal recessive (AR) cases have also been reported and are due to a gene mutation (18q) that encodes desmoglein 4 (DSG4), a situation that affects affinity for plakoglobin and alters hair shaft desmosomes [7].

Clinical diagnosis: The clinical picture includes diffuse hypotrichosis and short, fragile, and beaded hairs. Localized (occipital region) or generalized marked follicular hyperkeratosis may also be seen (Figure 1.1).

Optical microscopy: Alternating periodical beading (defect) and knots (normal hair shaft diameter) are characteristic aspects that may also be seen in dermoscopy (Figure 1.2). The hair shaft diameter is normal in the beaded segment of the hair shaft and the medulla is observed; these are not seen in the narrowed segments.

Scanning electron microscopy: Microscopic images are similar to those observed in optical microscopy; hair shaft fracture is evidenced in narrowed segments.

Trichoscopy: Dermoscopy is a useful tool for diagnosing hair shaft dysplasias. The typical "pearl necklace" image shows elliptical beading, regularly separated by narrowing segments where hair shaft fractures are usually observed. These findings are easily identified by dermoscopy— a simple method for a quick diagnosis [8,9] (Figure 1.3).

Histology: Intrafollicular hair shaft narrowing is observed.

TABLE 1.1

Classification of Hair Dysplasias

Dysplasias with Hair Fragility	Dysplasias with Little or No Hair Fragility
Monilethrix	Pili annulati
Pseudomonilethrix	Pseudopili annulati
Pili torti	Diffuse woolly hair
Menkes syndrome (kinky hair)	Woolly hair nevus
Trichorrexis invaginata (Netherton syndrome)	Acquired progressive kinking
Trichothiodystrophy	Diffuse partial woolly hair
Trichonodosis	Acquired partial curly hair
Distal trichorrhexis nodosa	Straight hair nevus
Proximal trichorrhexis nodosa	Pili canaliculi
Bubble hair	
Loose anagen hair	

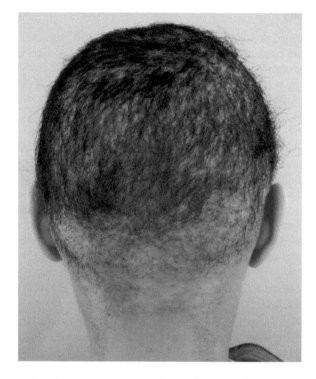

FIGURE 1.1   Monilethrix. Diffuse hypotrichosis in occipital region is characteristic.

Pseudomonilethrix

Pseudomonilethrix is a rare AD defect characterized by hair fragility. Localized or diffuse hypothicosis and fake knots (irregular hair shaft flattening) occur as the result of compulsive and frequent combing of the hair. Follicular hyperkeratosis is not observed. Individuals of different generations within the same family may be affected [10,11]. This condition may be associated with trichorrexis nodosa and bubble hair.

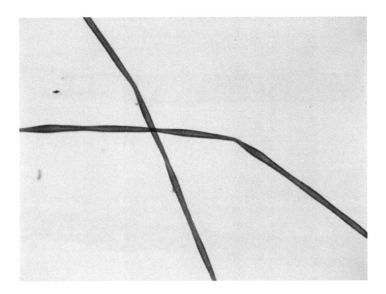

FIGURE 1.2   Typical beading with alternating knots and narrowed segments is observed.

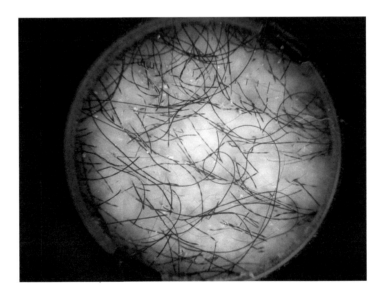

FIGURE 1.3   Elliptical beading with narrowed segments is seen on trichoscopy.

Genetics: Pseudomonilethrix is an AD defect. Specific genetic alterations have not been reported yet.

Clinical diagnosis: It is a familiar localized or diffuse hypotrichosis without follicular hyperkeratosis.

Optical microscopy: Rounded, normal appearing hairs with scarce and irregular oval or round nodules are present. Hair shaft narrowing is not observed (Figure 1.4).

Electron microscopy: What appear as nodules are actually flat segments of the hair shaft (Figure 1.5).

Trichoscopy: There are irregular distributed oval or round nodules without hair shaft narrowing segments and alternating of normal and wider segments of the hair shaft. No follicular hyperkeratosis is observed.

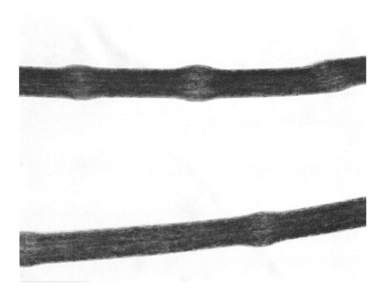

FIGURE 1.4   Pseudomonilethrix. Note round flattened nodules without hair shaft narrowing.

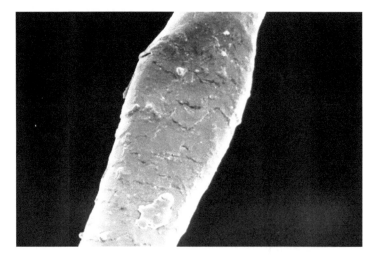

FIGURE 1.5   Hair shaft flattening is observed on scanning electron microscopy (SEM).

Acquired or Iatrogenic Pseudomonilethrix (Pseudopseudomonilethrix)

This defect is similar to pseudomonilethrix and arises from improper hair handling. It occurs when excessive pressure is applied to hair shafts during collection of samples from patients with monilethrix, woolly hair, and other conditions [12,13] (Figure 1.6). The same artifact is seen when a hair shaft is pressed between two slides (Figure 1.7).

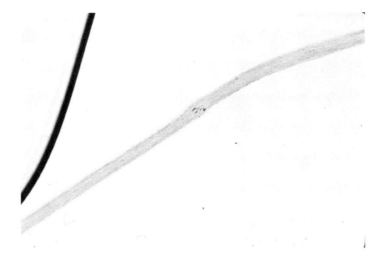

FIGURE 1.6   Acquired pseudomonilethrix. The artifact in dysplastic hair is due to excessive pressure from removing hair with fingers, forceps, or tweezers.

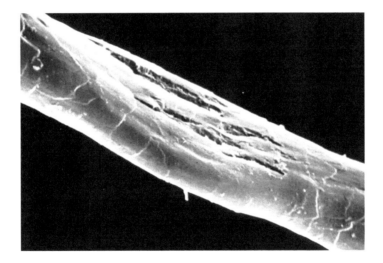

FIGURE 1.7   Another view of acquired pseudomonilethrix.

Pili Torti

This disease involves braided hair with periodic angles about its longitudinal axis. It is an AD or AR defect that may be isolated or associated with other diseases such as Beare-Stevenson, Bazex, Crandall, Björnstad, or type 2 congenital paronychia syndromes. Atypical pili torti associated with Menkes (kinky hair) syndrome and other hair dysplasias such as pili canaliculi and woolly hair has been observed [3]. Hair appears unusually bright due to light reflection and hypotrichosis may also be observed due to oblique fractures of the hair shafts (trichoclasis) [14]. Acquired and sporadic types are also recognized [15,16].

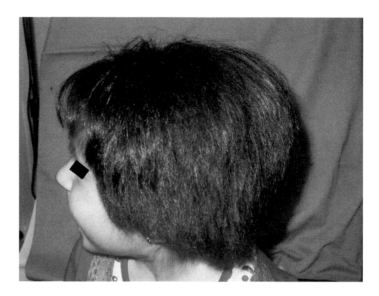

FIGURE 1.8   Pili torti. Abundant hairs with variable bright areas appearing like sequins.

Genetics: Mutation of *BSC1L* (Cr 2q34–36, 2q33) is responsible for malfunctioning of adenosine triphosphatase (ATPase) involved in mitochondrial complex III synthesis, a situation that leads to oxygen-reactive species that damage sensitive ear and hair follicle cells [17]. At least this is the case in Björnstad syndrome (AD) in which neurosensorial deafness and pili torti are observed [18]. More recently, this gene has been identified in the 2 Mb region between D2S2210 and D2S2244.

Mutation of the *ST14* gene (Cr 11q24.3–q.25) that encodes a protease (the matriptase type II transmembrane serine protease) has been identified in cases of pili torti associated with hypotrichosis and ichthyosis [19]. When associated with congenital hypotrichosis and juvenile macular dystrophy [20], the mutation has been identified in 16q22.1 [21]. Other mutations have been also identified in *CDH3*.

Clinical diagnosis: Patients usually have much hair that appears irregularly bright, depending on lighting conditions, and resembles sequins (Figure 1.8). It may be associated with localized hypotrichosis.

Optical microscopy: Braided hair with regular periodic angles is observed.

Electron microscopy: Images are similar to those observed in optical microscopy. Additionally, cuticle defects are found where steep angles occur (Figure 1.9).

Trichoscopy: Flattened hair shafts with turns at regular intervals are observed. In some cases, the defect is restricted only to a segment of the hair shaft [9]. These findings are observed more easily at ×70.

Biopsy: The same defect is observed in the hair follicles.

Associated conditions: Pili torti may be associated with nail dystrophy, ocular and teeth defects, follicular hyperkeratosis, and mental retardation.

Menkes Syndrome (Kinky Hair)

This is a recessive, sex-liked hereditary trait due to an alteration of intracellular copper use and transfer, a condition that leads to intestinal malabsorption of the metal and consequently to low levels of copper and ceruloplasmin in plasma and organs (brain, liver, bone, elastin, hair, and skin). This syndrome is complex and involves neurological manifestations associated with hypothermia, delay in psychomotor

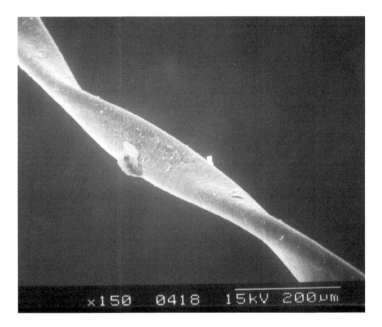

FIGURE 1.9   Braided hair with cuticle defects observed under scanning electron microscopy.

development, limb palsies, deafness, dwarfism, hernias, and other conditions [22,23]. Affected children show peculiar faces (e.g., partridge face profile) and scarce, fine, brittle, light hair. Death takes place quickly due to neurological complications. We recently reported a case of a newborn with Menkes syndrome and transitory neonatal erythroderma [24].

Genetics: Gene *ATP7A* encodes a transmembrane protein that controls cellular exit of copper. A mutation of this gene is responsible for multiple sclerosis (MS) and other conditions. The gene is located on chromosomes X (Xq21.1), 4, 9 (9q31–q32), 14, and 18 (18.26.0 cM) [25,26].

Clinical diagnosis: The characteristic patient is a newborn with a peculiar partridge face. Other features are convulsions, and fine, scarce, brittle, light hair (Figure 1.10).

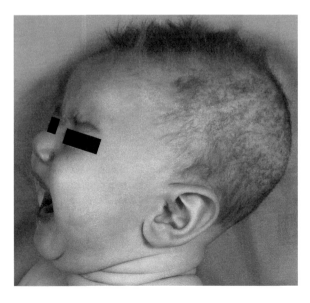

FIGURE 1.10   Menkes syndrome. Partridge face and poor dry hair are characteristic.

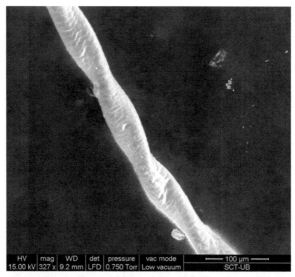

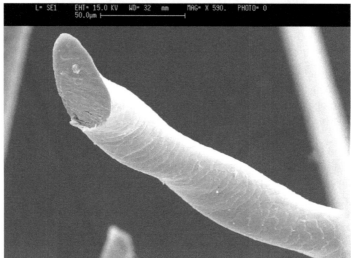

FIGURE 1.11   Atypical pili torti observed with scanning electron microscopy.

Optical microscopy: Kinky or polydysplastic hair: atypical irregular pili torti, monilethrix, and/or trichorrhexis nodosa.

Electron microscopy: Images are similar to those observed under optical microscopy (Figure 1.11). Defects of the hair cuticle are also observed, especially cuticle cells with saw aspects.

X-ray microanalysis: Low copper and sulfur contents have been reported.

Trichoscopy: Hair diameter is variable. Some segments are narrow while others look irregularly flat and twisted around their axes (atypical pili torti), a condition that may be similar to monilethrix. Irregular or atypical trichorrhesis may be found frequently.

Trichorrhexis Invaginata (Netherton Syndrome)

Trichorrhexis invaginata includes both ballooning distortions of the hair shafts and chaliced deformations of the proximal hair shaft areas. This characteristic alteration gives a hair shaft a bamboo cane appearance; therefore, this hair dysplasia is also known as "bamboo hair." It is a specific anomaly considered a marker for Netherton syndrome, which is an AR genodermatosis observed more frequently in females. It may be associated with trichorrhesis invaginata, atopy, ichthyosis linearis circumflexa, erythroderma ichthyosiforme congenital, and ichthyosis vulgaris [3,27].

Genetics: Various gene mutations have been reported: *kallikrein, corneodesmosin, desmochollin 1, desmoglein 1, transglutaminase 1, filaggrin, serine peptidase inhibitor* and *SPINK5* that encodes LEKTI, a serine protease inhibitor (5q.32), and *NETS* (5q.32) [28,29].

Clinical diagnosis: Characteristically, the affected individual is a female with ichthyosis linearis circumflexa (plaques with double squamous borders), atopy, and diffuse hypotrichosis (scarce and brittle hair) (Figure 1.12). Associated conditions are ichthyosis vulgaris or erythroderma ichthyosiforme congenita. Trichothiodystrophy may also be associated to ichthyosis, a condition that should be ruled out.

Optical microscopy: Bamboo hair (trichorrhesis invaginata) is a typical image, It is a ballooning deformity of the hair shaft that lies in a proximal chaliced-shaped area. Eyebrows and eyelashes may be also affected.

Electron microscopy: The images are similar to those observed by an optical microscope (Figure 1.13). Hair shaft distal ends may appear as a golf poles due to hair fractures at the knots of trichorrhexis invaginata.

Trichoscopy: Hairs are fractured at the nodules or knots where a shaft appears as a bamboo cane knot. Typical aspects are chaliced shapes of the proximal ends and ballooning distortions of the distal parts of knots. Distal ends of hair shafts show a golf pole aspect due to local fracture [30,31].

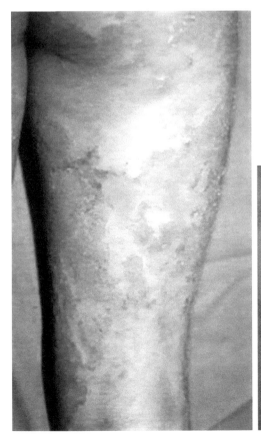
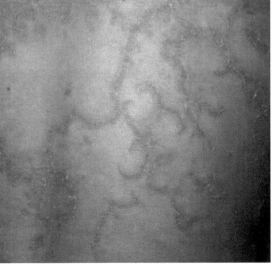

FIGURE 1.12   Trichorrhexis invaginata (Netherton disease). Girls with scarce, poor, dry hair usually present with ichthyosis linearis circumflexa characterized by squamous double borders. (Courtesy of Prof. P. de Unamuno.)

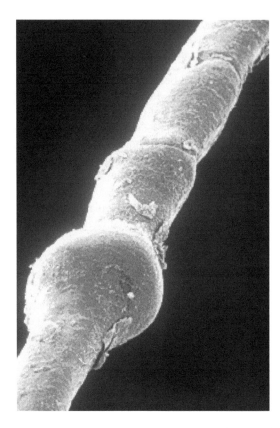

FIGURE 1.13   Typical "bamboo hair" with proximal dilatation of the hair shaft into chalice-shape distortion and distal ballooning alteration.

Trichothiodystrophy

Trichothiodystrophy (TTD) is a complex syndrome caused by low levels of sulfur compounds in the hair that lead to a specific dysplasia known as trichodystrophic hair [1,3,32]. The syndrome is associated with other clinical findings such as a delay in psychomotor development, ichthyosis, onycodystrophy, microdolicocephalia, photosensitivity, and other defects [33,34]. Some variations of the syndrome include BIDS (Brittle hair, Intellectual impairment + Decreased fertility and Short stature or Amish brittle hair syndrome or TTD type D), IBIDS (Ichthyosis or Tay syndrome or TTD type E), PIBIDS (Phosensitivity or TTD type F), SIBIDS (+osteoSclerosis, ONMRS or Itin syndrome), and syndromes of Sabinas (TTD type B, with nail dystrophy) and Pollit (TTD type C, + neonatal retardation). The term TTD type A is reserved for when only the isolated congenital hair defect is present.

> **Genetics:** Mutations of TTD, ERCC2, C7orf11, ERCC3, GTF2H5, XPC, and GTF2H4 genes localized in 19q13.2–q13.3, 19q13.3, 7p14.1, 2q21, 6q25.3, 3p25, and 6p21.3, respectively, have been reported [37–39].
>
> **Clinical diagnosis:** The affected individual is a newborn with congenital ichthyosis, scarce, short, and brittle hair, and a characteristic face: microdolicocephalia and pleasant appearance (Figure 1.14). Other clinical findings may include mental retardation, growth delay, onycodystrophy (nail striae), and photosensitivity [33].

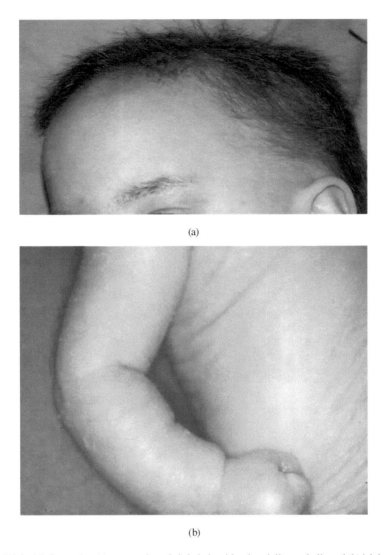

FIGURE 1.14   Trichothiodystrophy: (a) scarce, short, brittle hair with microdolicocephalia and (b) ichthyosis.

Optical microscopy: Flat hair appears with typical transverse and clean transversal fractures (trichoschisis); see Figure 1.15a.

Polarized light: Alternating light and dark bands in the hair presenting a typical spotted tiger-like surface are observed; see Figure 1.15b.

Scanning electron microscopy: Completely rigid flat hairs that resemble tapes are observed. Trichoschisis with a clean fracture is pathognomonic. The hair surface shows longitudinal crests and cuticle defects (Figure 1.16).

X-ray microanalysis: Sulfur content is lower than 50% (Figure 1.17).

Amino acid chromatography: Hair-sulfured amino acids are clearly lowered.

Trichoscopy: Dermoscopy is not characteristic except for the trichoschisis [40]. Hair shafts may also show weaving contours and non-homogeneous structures such as grains of sand, alternating dark and light bands, and spotted tiger-like surfaces.

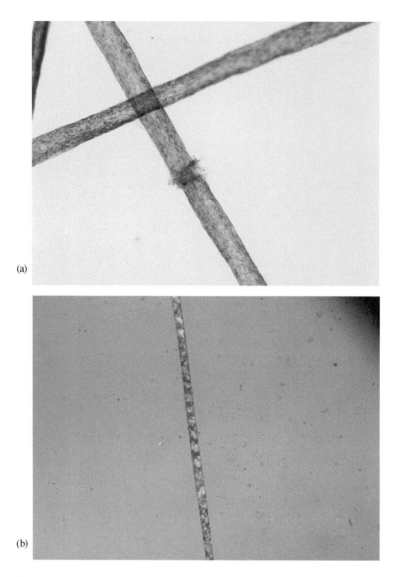

(a)

(b)

FIGURE 1.15   Trichothiodystrophy: (a) Flat hair with typical transverse fractures (trichoschisis) and (b) characteristic spotted tiger tail-like appearance.

Trichonodosis

This is a frequent but rarely diagnosed hair dysplasia in which true knots are observed along the hair shafts. It may be suspected when hair shafts show angles and abruptly change their directions [2,41]. This condition is more frequently observed in individuals with curly hair in association with local trauma, scraping maneuvers, and tics [42]. It may be found in the armpit and genitalia in association with pediculosis and acarophobia. How the double or even more complex knots are originated is not yet completely understood.

> **Clinical diagnosis:** Trichonodosis usually occurs as an isolated finding. Suspicions may arise when a hair abruptly changes its direction due to a true knot.
> **Optical microscopy:** A simple, double, or even complex true knot ("tie knot") is observed (Figure 1.18).

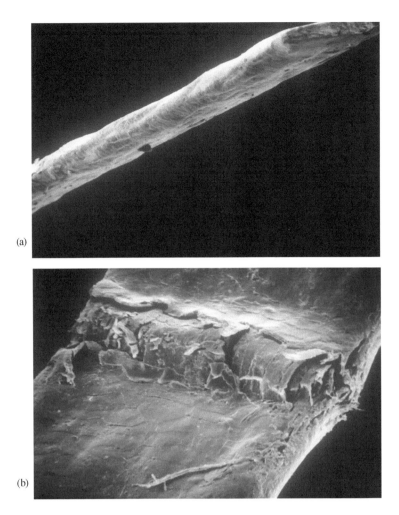

(a)

(b)

FIGURE 1.16 Trichothiodystrophy: Scanning electron micrographs of (a) flat hair resembling tape and (b) initial trichoschisis.

Scanning electron microscopy: Similar images to those observed by optical microscopy are seen. Amplification may reveal cuticle defects in the true knot area (Figure 1.19).

Trichoscopy: A simple, double, or complex true knot is observed. Sometimes a "tie knot" or a "sailor knot" is observed in dermoscopy.

Distal Trichorrhexis Nodosa

Trichorrhexis nodosa is defined as the presence of nodules of fracture on hair shafts. Clinical findings differ, depending whether the fracture occurs proximally or distally in the shaft [2,42]. Alopecia is observed only in the former case.

Distal trichorrhexis nodosa is an acquired diffuse condition more frequently observed in long hair and is caused by external physical and/or chemical factors and weathering in predisposed individuals.

Clinical diagnosis: This disorder is more frequently seen in young long-haired women who are exposed to physical and chemical factors related to esthetic procedures. Hair usually shows little balls (nodules of fracture) at the distal ends. Hair shaft breaks at these little balls and final ends of the hair shafts bifurcate (trichoptilosis). Patients normally complain of no hair growth

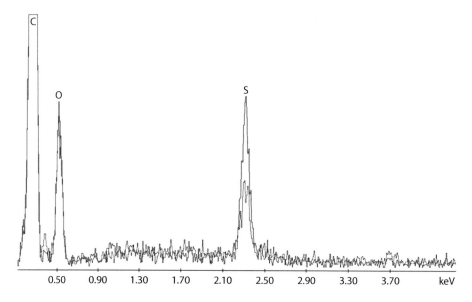

FIGURE 1.17   Low sulfur content revealed by x-ray microanalysis. The red spectrum corresponds to a control normal hair and the brown one to the patient.

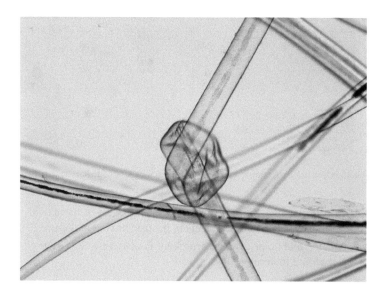

FIGURE 1.18   Trichonodosis. A knot in a hair shaft may be simple, double, or more complex.

and haircuts are not needed because the hair breaks off easily when manipulated minimally (Figure 1.20).

Pull test is positive (Saboureaud's sign) and hair easily breaks off at the points where little balls appear. The examiner usually finds short segments of distal broken hair shafts.

Optical microscopy: Fractures at nodules are clearly seen and both sides of nodules show chipping aspects of the cortex (Figure 1.21). When two segments of hair are pulled apart, both hair shaft ends look like a brush. Bifurcated hair endings (trichoptilosis) resulting from external factors are also seen. Trichorrhesis nodosa may also be observed in other hair dysplasias, mainly in Menkes syndrome.

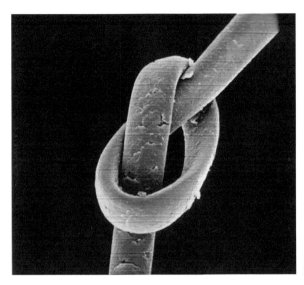

FIGURE 1.19   True knot with cuticle defects observed by scanning electron microscopy.

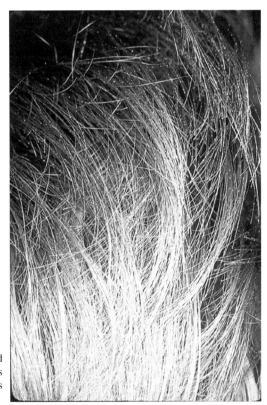

FIGURE 1.20   Distal trichorrhexis nodosa. Long-haired individuals are affected more frequently. The hair shows little balls that appear as dust spots and bifurcated endings (trichoptilosis).

Electron microscopy: Altered or absent cuticles are observed along with typical images of trichorrhexis nodosa and trichoptilosis. The cuticle and cortex show small spalling areas close to the fracture zones at the nodules under both transmission and scanning electron microscopy [43,44].

Trichoscopy: Nodules where fractures take place are easily seen. At higher magnification, cortex fibers are also seen at the fracture points. At lower magnification, lighter nodules and slits along

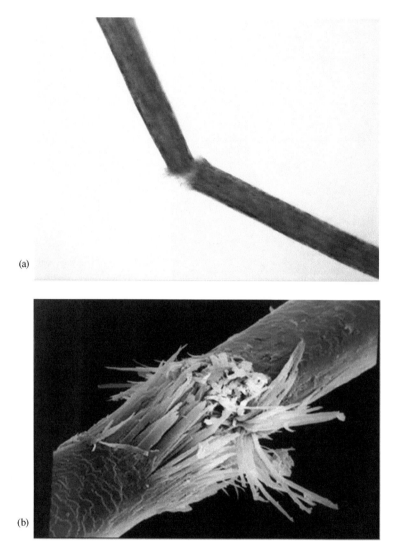

FIGURE 1.21   Trichorrexis nodosa: (a) Fracture of hair shaft at nodule, with both sides of the nodule showing open spalling of cortex; (b) SEM.

the hair shafts are observed. Hair endings look like brushes. Dermoscopy is a useful and fast tool for diagnosing trichorrhesis nodosa [9,40].

Treatment: It is mandatory for patients to avoid constant hair treatments such as obsessive combing and brushing. They should also avoid exposure to heat, dust, wind, salt, and repetitive physical–chemical and intense cosmetic treatments. Finally, haircuts are advisable.

Proximal Trichorrhexis Nodosa

The morphological defect is the same one observed in the distal variant; however, the proximal variation is a more complex condition since trichorrhexis nodosa and trichoptilosis repetitively alternate in the very same hairs [45]. Proximal trichorrhexis nodosa is seen more frequently in black people who may show hypotrichosis in the scalp, beard, mustache, and other anatomical regions. It may be a hereditary disorder [46], a marker of congenital argininosuccinic aciduria [47], or trichohepatoenteric syndrome [48].

Genetics: Trichorrhesis nodosa associated with Pollit syndrome is a variant of trichothiodystrophy without photosensitivity. Gene mutations have been reported in *C7ORF11* and *TFIIH*.

Clinical diagnosis: Alopecic hairs may be found in areas of the scalp, beard, mustache, and pubis. Hairs look short and broken; their endings show little balls appearing like dust spots (Figure 1.22). Proximal trichorrhexis nodosa may be confused easily with trichotillomania and bubble hair.

Optical microscopy: Typical images of trichorrhexis nodosa and trichoptilosis are observed (Figure 1.23).

Electron microscopy: Complex images of trichorrhexis nodosa and trichoptilosis are frequently observed in the same area and associated with cuticle defects under both transmission and scanning electron microscopic examinations (Figure 1.24).

Trichoscopy: As stated in the above section, dermoscopy shows complex images of some nodules of fractures in the same hair shaft, always close to the scalp.

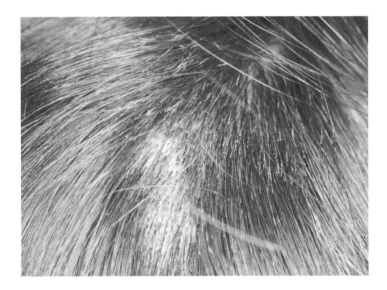

FIGURE 1.22 Proximal trichorrhexis nodosa. Hypotrichotic area with short broken hairs is seen.

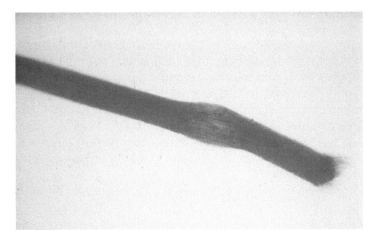

FIGURE 1.23 Typical image of trichorrhexis nodosa and hair shaft fracture at nodule with spalling of cortex distally.

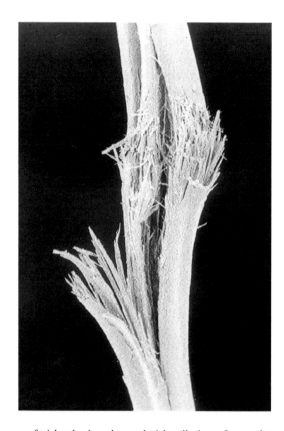

FIGURE 1.24   Complex images of trichorrhexis nodosa and trichoptilosis are frequently seen.

Bubble Hair

This acquired hair dysplasia is caused by air bubbles trapped within the hair—a situation in predisposed individuals that may be due to intense hair drying [49,50]. It is more common in women who show localized hypotrichotic plaques. Dry heating may widen hair medullae and cause cortex dilatations that appear as bubbles on the hair shaft surfaces. The hair shafts may break off at their widest ballooning segments.

Clinical diagnosis: This condition may be suspected in women who exhibit sudden hypotrichotic plaques with short, broken hairs, and a fractured end appearance is observed. Predisposed individuals usually use intense hair drying at close range.

Optical microscopy: The typical image is a ballooning hair shaft surface with trapped air bubbles.

Scanning electron microscopy: Swollen or ballooning aspects of the hair shafts due to cortex dilatations are seen. Superficial orifices and fissures may be also present. Final hair endings show an image resembling Gruyère cheese due to bubbles or cavitations. Bubbles may also be found between cuticle layers [51].

Trichoscopy: Confluent ballooning or ballooning at different points of a hair shaft is observed (Figure 1.25).

Treatment: It is mandatory for patients to avoid the cause of this condition: intense and frequent hair drying.

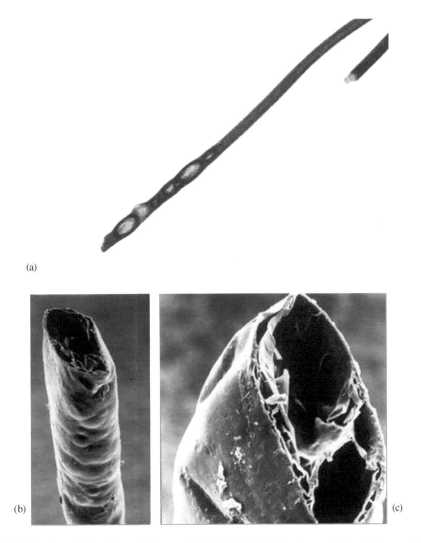

(a)

(b)

(c)

FIGURE 1.25 Ballooning of hair shafts at different points in bubble hair is clearly revealed by trichoscopy (a) and scanning electron microscopy (b) and (c).

Loose Anagen Hair

Loose anagen hair is a dysplasia due to lack of adhesion of hair shafts to hair follicles. It is more frequently observed in young blonde girls whose hair is lost easily and causes no pain when pulled [52,53]. Affected hair shows a ruffling aspect in intrafollicular areas.

Genetics: Gene mutations have been reported in *SHOC2* and *KRT75* [54,55]. The former encodes a rich leucine-containing protein that participates in protein–protein interactions during cascade activation of kinases (Ras proteins, extracellular signal-regulated kinase [ERK], mitogen-activated protein [MAP] kinase). This mutation is responsible for Noonan-like syndrome with loose anagen hair. *KRT75* encodes a family of type 2 keratins that participate in formation of hair and nails. Genes have been identified in 10q.25 and 12q.13.

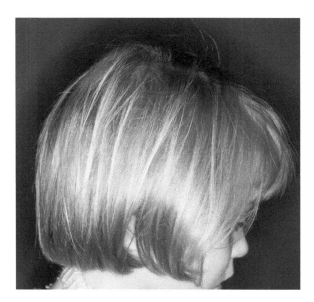

FIGURE 1.26 Loose anagen hair. This dysplasia is observed in 3- to 6-year-old blonde girls who show spontaneous, easy, painless hair loss, especially when hair is only minimally pulled. The condition improves over time.

> **Clinical diagnosis:** Loose anagen hair is observed more frequently in 3- to 6-year-old blonde girls. Hair is lost easily and without pain when pulled. Patients report spontaneous, diffuse hair loss, especially when it is pulled with minimum force. Haircuts are not necessary because hair grows only to a certain length (Figure 1.26). Reported familial cases are rare and may be associated with some ectodermic dysplasias [56]. Other associations include Moyamoya disease with Noonan-like syndrome [57].
>
> **Optical microscopy:** Observations are twisted anagen roots and proximal cuticle ruffling (Figure 1.27).
>
> **Scanning electron microscopy:** Twisted anagen roots with cuticle ruffling limited to the intrafollicular portions are observed. Images may also reveal pili canaliculi.
>
> **Trichoscopy:** Twisted anagen roots with cuticle ruffling may be observed. Recently, rectangular granular structures that represent empty follicles have also been described.
>
> **Prognosis:** No treatment has been reported. However, the condition may improve spontaneously over time.

Pili Annulati (Ringed Hair)

Pili annulati or "Morse alphabet" hair is perhaps the only condition other than bubble hair that affects the hair medulla that shows alternating dilatations of the medulla that gives the hair shaft a ringed appearance. Alternating dark and bright bands are observed in the hair shaft due to trapped air in the cortex and medulla (dark bands) and keratin distortions that diffuse incident light (bright bands) [1,2]. Pili annulati is an AD trait or sporadic condition that affects individuals with thick normal-appearing hair. In both cases, it is an esthetic condition that may be accepted by an affected individual. Delays in hair growth and low cystine content that may lead to altered formation of the microfibril complex have been reported.

> **Genetics:** The gene responsible for this hair dysplasia has been reported to be in region 9.2 cM of chromosome 12q between *D12S367* and *D12S1723* [58].
>
> **Clinical diagnosis:** This hair condition affects young females with thick normal-appearing hair that shows alternating dark and bright bands that may resemble sequins as in pili torti and can be observed without a light source (Figure 1.28).

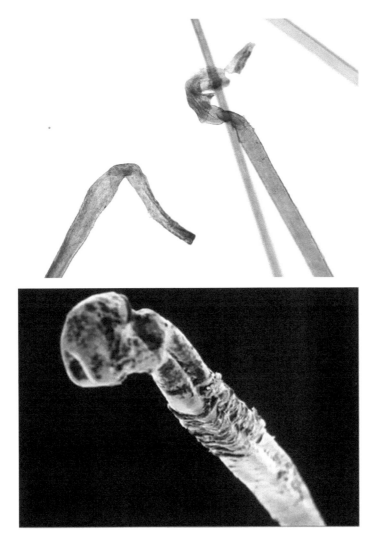

FIGURE 1.27   Loose anagen hair. Twisted anagen hair with cuticle ruffling is observed.

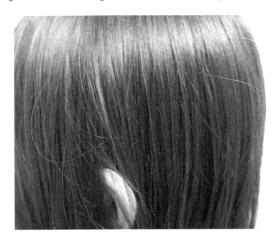

FIGURE 1.28   Pili annulati. Alternating dark and light bands are seen in ringed hair in females with thick, bright, normal-appearing hair.

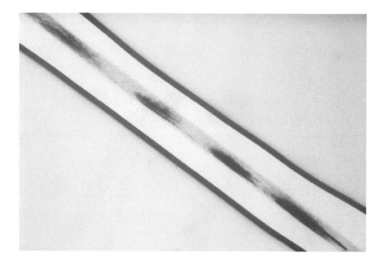

FIGURE 1.29   Regular alternating dark and light bands are clearly seen.

Optical microscopy: Regular alternating dark (cavitations with trapped air in the medullae) and bright bands are seen (Figure 1.29). Polarized light clearly reveals these bands.

Electron microscopy: Alternating dark and bright bands are observed in transmission and scanning electron microscopy. As in optical microscope images, dark bands correspond to cavitations in the medullae and thinner cortex. Cuticles show small cavitations that lead to increased permeability and trap air within the hair [59,60].

Trichoscopy: Light bands correspond to trapped air in cavitations in contrast to optical microscopy images in which they appear as dark bands. Individuals with normal thick hair may show light bands known as pseudopili annulati that affect less than 50% of hair width [9].

Pseudopili Annulati

This condition is considered a variation of normal hair appearance in which an optical or physical defect leads to the presence of bands like those observed in pili annulati, but without hair fragility. Bands result from light reflected at a straight angle by flat twisted segments of the hair shaft that act as small mirrors [61,62].

Clinical diagnosis: Children with dark or golden hair show alternating dark and bright bands. No hereditary cases have been reported to date.

Optical microscopy: Bands are only observed if light is shone perpendicularly on the longitudinal axes of the hair.

Polarized light microscopy: This tool reveals only variability in hair shaft diameters without alternating bands, in contrast to findings in true pili annulati.

Scanning electron microscopy: Hair shaft cross-sections are elliptical while long axes show wider and narrower segments. Moreover, alternating 30- to 40-degree twisting in two different directions is observed [62].

Trichoscopy: Variations in hair shaft diameter are observed. No alternating bands (as seen in true pili annulati) are present.

Generalized Woolly Hair

Woolly hair is the presence of curly, flat, thinner-than-normal hair in Caucasians. It is different from the hair of black individuals that is normally flat and curly. Three groups of woolly hair are recognized currently: (1) generalized or diffuse woolly hair (congenital AD or AR), (2) woolly hair nevus (congenital, localized or multifocal, possibly associated with other conditions), and (3) acquired woolly hair (progressive curly hair, mainly partial and diffuse). The generalized or diffuse variant rarely occurs and may affect the entire scalp. The disorder may be associated with altered keratinization and eye, teeth, and bone defects, among other conditions [2,63,64].

> **Genetics:** AD variants are due to a mutation of *KTR74* (12q13, 20.91 MB between *D12S1301* and *D12S1610*) [65]. AR variants are caused by mutations in *P2RY5* (13q14.2–q14.3), *LIPH* (3q27–q28), and *LAH2* (3q27–q28) (66). In Naxos disease, woolly hair is associated with cardiomyopathy and keratoderma of the palms and soles and is caused by the mutation of the *plakoglobin* gene (17q.21) [67].
>
> **Clinical diagnosis:** Children normally show very thin, soft, curly hair that resembles wool. Hair has low density and the scalp can be seen easily through the hair (Figure 1.30). Hair fragility may lead to some hypotrichotic areas. This condition should be differentiated from uncombable hair, a distinctive dysplasia with which it has been confused in medical literature.
>
> **Optical microscopy:** Images reveal thin curly hairs that form small balls.
>
> **Histopathology:** Normal quantities of groups of miniaturized anagen hair follicles are visible.
>
> **Scanning electron microscopy:** Very flat, noodle-like, curly hairs with oval cross-sections are seen (Figure 1.31). Other findings may be isolated twisting and pili canaliculi.
>
> **Trichoscopy:** Rudnicka et al. [40] reported cyclical short wavy hair that recalls a characteristic "moving snake" image. Also seen are broken hairs whose fragility is caused by longitudinal twisting (Figure 1.32).

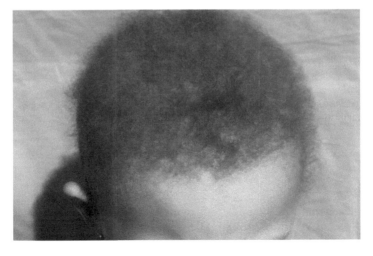

FIGURE 1.30 Characteristically diffuse woolly hair presenting in a child with very soft, curly hair. The reduced density enables an examiner to directly observe the scalp.

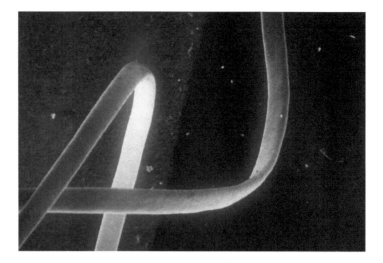

FIGURE 1.31   Hair shafts in woolly hair are very flat, like noodles, and have oval cross-sections.

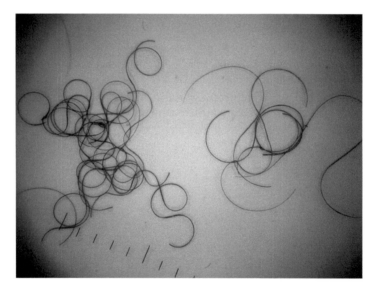

FIGURE 1.32   On trichoscopy, woolly hair appears cyclical, short, and wavy and resembles a moving snake; longitudinal twisting increases fragility and leads to broken hairs.

Woolly Hair Nevus

This is a localized, congenital, non-familial variant of woolly hair. It can be isolated or multifocal and represents the most common form of curly and kinky hair syndromes [68]. Nearly 50% of cases are associated with melanocytic nevus or epidermal nevus in the same affected area or on the head [69]. Other alterations may include ocular problems (cataracts, retinal dysplasia, persistent or pupilar membrane), teeth defects and gingivitis, growth and speaking delays, and congenital triangular alopecia [70]. No genetic findings have been reported.

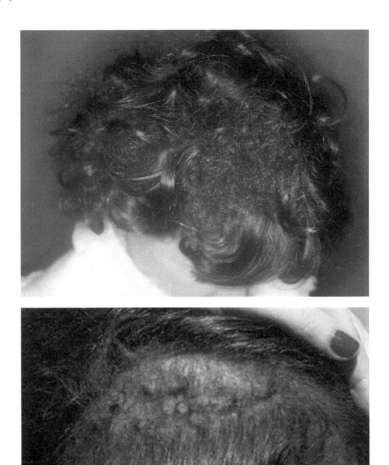

FIGURE 1.33 Woolly hair nevus exhibits one or more areas of woolly, fine, thin, curly hair surrounded by normal-appearing hair.

Clinical diagnosis: One or more areas of woolly, curly, thin, light hair surrounded by normal hair are observed. Isolated plaques are the most common presentations; multifocality is seldom reported (Figure 1.33). Melanocytic and epidermal nevi may be present in the same affected area or on other areas of the head.

Optical microscopy: Hair looks very thin, flat, and light and forms balls. Cross-sections are oval.

Histopathology: Areas of grouped miniaturized anagen follicles are observed.

Scanning electron microscopy: The hair appears flat and curly; cross-sections are oval. Longitudinal twisting and channels along the axes are also observed. Fewer cuticle layers than normal may also be seen.

Trichoscopy: The same findings revealed for generalized woolly hair are found in circumscribed areas.

Treatment: Because woolly hair nevus is a localized hair dysplasia, surgery is a therapeutic alternative to be considered.

Acquired and Progressive Kinking of Hair

Acquired and progressive kinking of hair is an acquired non-familial variant of woolly hair that frequently affects male teenagers. Locks of hair become curly and kinky and the condition slowly but progressively affects the entire scalp. No external factors have been identified and the condition slowly progresses to androgenetic alopecia [71–73]. A localized variant known as whisker hair nevus or circumscribed symmetric allotrichia has been reported. Systemic retinoids have been cited as a possible cause of acquired and progressive kinky hair. No genetic findings have been reported yet.

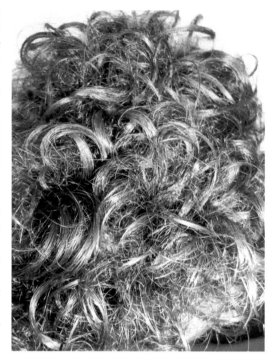

FIGURE 1.34   Acquired progressive kinking of hair usually affects male teenagers. Multiple locks appear curly and kinky.

> **Clinical diagnosis:** Typical patients are male teenagers who show locks of acquired thin kinky hair (Figure 1.34).
>
> **Optical microscopy:** Curly, flat hair that appears oval in cross-sections is visible.
>
> **Histopathology:** A cross-section shows oval hair follicles (Figure 1.35).
>
> **Scanning electron microscopy:** Affected hair is thin and curly and appears flat, like noodles. Cross-section reveals diffuse or localized oval hairs as in congenital woolly hair (Figure 1.36).
>
> **Trichoscopy:** The same findings are observed as in generalized or diffuse woolly hair.

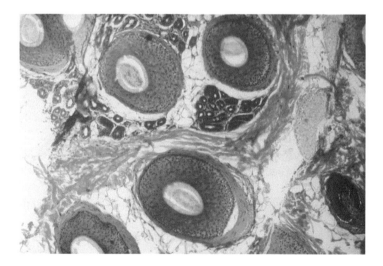

FIGURE 1.35   Cross-section shows oval hair follicles.

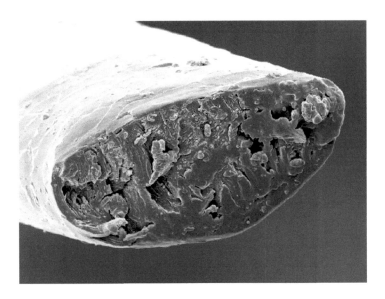

FIGURE 1.36   Affected hairs are flat, like woolly hairs, with oval cross-sections.

Diffuse Partially Woolly Hair

This is a new variant of acquired kinking of hair that involves individual and isolated kinking; usually a single curly kinky hair is observed among 10 or 12 normal hairs. The disorder may be sporadic or familial. No external factors have been identified and most affected individuals are children or teenagers [74,75].

Genetics: An AD trait may be related to a mutation of *KRT74* (12q.13) described above in the generalized woolly hair section.

Clinical diagnosis: This disorder is observed in children and teenagers with isolated curly and kinking of hair that stands out from normal hair.

Optical microscopy: Affected hair looks flat, curly, and oval in cross-section.

Histopathology: Anagen curved hair follicles among normal-appearing follicles are observed.

Scanning electron microscopy: Affected hair is thinner and flatter than normal hair and appears oval on cross-section. Twisting and longitudinal channels may also be present.

Trichoscopy: Affected hair is flat and curly. Findings are similar to those above described for woolly hair nevus.

Acquired Partially Curly Hair

This is a partial and acquired variant of kinking that affects isolated hairs in the scalp and may be confused with diffuse partially woolly hair. This is a non-familial condition that affects only the distal part of the hair shaft, improves over time, and may be a response to external factors such as environmental conditions or cosmetic procedures [76].

Clinical diagnosis: The typical case is a young woman with isolated curly hairs surrounded by normal hairs (Figure 1.37). This is a sporadic and acquired condition, which differentiates it from diffuse partially woolly hair.

Optical microscopy: Affected hair is thinner, flatter, and curly only distally.

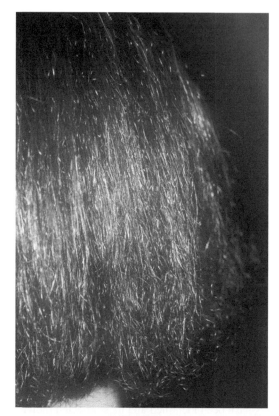

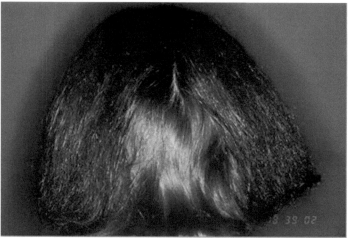

FIGURE 1.37   In acquired partially curly hair, children or teenagers exhibit isolated curly hairs in distal parts of hair shafts.

Scanning electron microscopy: Affected hair is flatter, thinner, and oval in cross-section. Characteristically, hair is normal in its proximal portions but acquires a thinner curly aspect in the distal parts of the hair shafts.

Trichoscopy: The condition displays the same findings seen in woolly hair nevus but only in isolated affected hairs that appear less curly.

Treatment: Hair conditioners may help. Avoidance of weathering and aggressive cosmetic treatments is mandatory.

Straight Hair Nevus

This disorder has been described as the inverse image of woolly hair nevus. It is characterized by a delimited area with straight hair locks surrounded by curly hairs [77]. In the few cases reported, the condition is linked to a local keratinization disorder associated with ichthyosis or epidermal nevus [78] and has also been reported in a patient with straight hair [79]. No genetic changes have been discovered.

Clinical diagnosis: One or more locks of straight hair are observed and they are surrounded characteristically by curly hair. However, the disorder has been found in individuals with only straight hair but variable hair diameters and associated with local epidermal defects.

Histopathology: In the only case that we reported, we noted hyperplasia of the sebaceous glands that gave a yellowish discoloration to the affected skin in an 8-year-old child.

Optical and electron microscopy: We observed minimal channels along the longitudinal axis.

X-ray microanalysis: No findings have been reported.

Trichoscopy: It is the inverse image of woolly hair; affected hair in this case appears straight.

Comment: Straight hair nevus has been reported to be associated with ichthyosis histryx and warty plaques of the affected skin independent of ethnic origin. Another plausible theory is that this condition corresponds to hair mosaicism or a hair follicle disorder induced by the affected skin and is not an individual and distinctive hair disease.

Uncombable Hair (Pili Canaliculi)

This syndrome is characterized by dry, light, scoured hair in children or teenagers with thick hair and locks in different directions that make the hair impossible to comb or style [80,81]. The disorder is also known as "spun glass hair." It is a sporadic or familial AD or AR condition [82]. It generally affects children with straight uncombable hair but has also been reported in young curly-haired individuals. Localized variants have also been reported. The common finding in all cases is the presence of pili canaliculi. However, pili canaliculi may also be found in ectodermal dysplasias, other hair dysplasias, and most cases of loose anagen hair.

Genetics: No genetic changes have been reported. However, in Rapp-Hodgkin syndrome (anhidrotic ectodermal dysplasia and cleft lip and/or palate), sometimes associated with pili canalicula, the mutation has been identified in *TP63* (3q.27) [83].

Clinical diagnosis: The disorder is seen in children or teenagers who show dry, lusterless hair that cannot be combed and it may be familial (Figure 1.38).

Optical microscopy: Channels beside hair shafts are observed easily by adjusting the micrometer (Figure 1.39). If a hair has a medulla, it is impossible to see the channel.

Histopathology: A biopsy is seldom required. Inner sheath adhesions and hair shaft twisting are observed [84].

Scanning electron microscopy: One or more channels are observed along the longitudinal axes of hair shafts and are definitive for the diagnosis (Figure 1.40). Depending on the number of channels, the cross-section of a hair shaft may show a kidney-like, triangular, square, or irregular shape [85].

Trichoscopy: Flattening and longitudinal channels are observed along the hair shaft axes, while cross-sections of the hairs show a kidney-like or triangular shape.

Treatment: Spontaneous improvement over time has been reported. Zinc pyrithione shampoo may improve hair due to rebound fat effect.

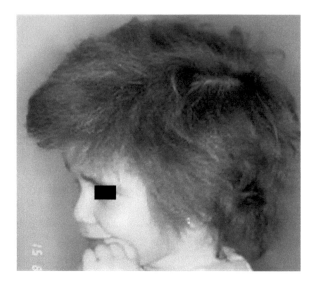

FIGURE 1.38   Pili canaliculi affects children and young individuals with dry, lusterless, uncombable hair.

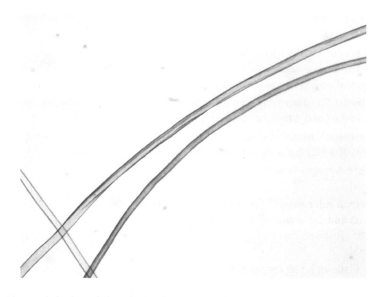

FIGURE 1.39   Characteristic channel along the longitudinal axis of hair shaft is observed.

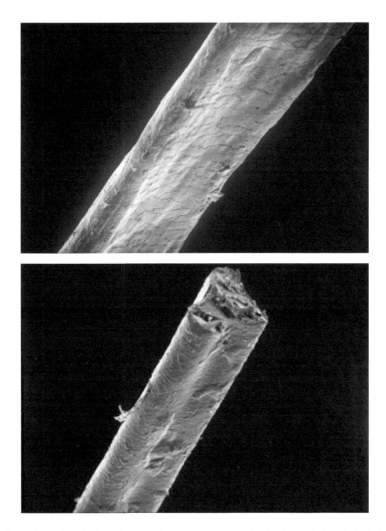

FIGURE 1.40 Deep channels and triangular or oval cross-sections are clearly observed along hair shafts.

REFERENCES

1. Camacho-Martínez F and Ferrando J. Hair shaft dysplasias. *Int J Dermatol* 27: 71–80, 1988.
2. Camacho FM, Tosti A, Randall VA, and Price VH. *Montagna Trichology*. Madrid: Aula Médica, 2016.
3. Van Neste D. Dysplasies pilaires congénitales: conduite á tenir et intérét de diverses méthodes de diagnostic. *Ann Dermatol Venerol* 116: 251–263, 1989.
4. De Berker DAR, Ferguson DJP, and Dawber RPR. Monilethrix: a clinicopathological illustration of a cortical defect. *Br J Dermatol* 128: 327–331, 1993.
5. Ferrando J, Fontarnau R, Castells-Mas A et al. Sequential study of the transversal fracture formation of the hair in monilethrix and trichorrhexis nodosa. *J Cutan Pathol* 8: 165, 1981.
6. Ferrando J, Galve J, Torres-Puente M et al. Monilethrix: a new family with the novel mutation in *KRT81* gene. *Int J Trichol* 4: 53–55, 2012.
7. Zlotogorski A, Marek D, Horev L et al. An autosomal recessive form of monilethrix is caused by mutations in *DSG4*: clinical overlap with localized autosomal recessive hypotrichosis. *J Invest Dermatol* 126: 1292–1296, 2006.
8. Ferrándiz L, Moreno D, Peral L et al. Tricoscopia. *Piel* 296: 1–7, 2011.

9. Miteva M and Tosti A. Dermoscopy of hair shaft disorders. *J Am Acad Dermatol* 68: 473–481, 2013.
10. Bentley-Phillips B and Bayles MA. A previously undescribed hereditary hair anomaly (pseudomonilethrix). *Br J Dermatol* 89: 1591–1567, 1973.
11. Bentley-Phillips B, Bayles MA, and Grace HJ. Pseudo-monilethrix: further family studies. *Humangenetik* 25: 331–337, 1974.
12. Ferrando J, Fontarnau R, and Hausmann G. Is pseudomonilethrix an artifact? *Int J Dermatol* 29: 380–381, 1990.
13. Zitelli JA. Pseudomonilethrix: an artifact. *Arch Dermatol*. 122: 688–690, 1986.
14. Marayuma T, Toyoda M, Kanei A et al. Pathogenesis in pili torti: morphological study. *J Dermatol Sci Suppl*. S5–S12, 1994.
15. Kurwa AR and Abdel-Aziz AHM. Pili torti: congenital and acquired. *Acta Dermatovenereol* 53: 585–588, 1973.
16. Lyon JB and Dawber RPR. A sporadic case of dystrophic pili torti. *Br J Dermatol* 96: 197–201, 1977.
17. BCS1L BCS1-like (*S. cerevisiae*) [*Homo sapiens*] Gene ID 617, updated November 8, 2010. http://www.ncbi.nlm.nih.gov/gene617
18. Petit A, Dontenville MM, Bardon CB et al. Pili torti with congenital deafness (Bjornstad syndrome): report of three cases in one family, suggesting autosomal dominant transmission. *Clin Exp Dermatol* 18: 94–95, 1993.
19. Hinson JT, Fantin VR, Schönberger J et al. Missense mutations in the *BCS1L* gene as a cause of Bjornstad syndrome. *New Engl J Med* 356: 809–819, 2007.
20. McGowan KM and Coulombe PA. Keratin 17 expression in the hard epithelial context of the hair and nail and its relevance for the pachyonychia congenita phenotype. *J Invest Dermatol* 114: 1101–1107, 2000.
21. Basel-Vanagaite L, Attia R, Ishida-Yamamoto A et al. Autosomal recessive ichthyosis with hypotrichosis caused by a mutation in *ST14* encoding type II transmembrane serine protease matriptase. *Am J Hum Genet* 80: 467–477, 2007.
22. Danks DM, Cartwright E, Stevens BJ et al. Menkes' kinky hair disease: future definition of the defect in cooper transport. *Science* 179: 1140–1142, 1973.
23. Díaz Pérez JL, Rúa MJ, Prats J et al. Enfermedad de Menkes. Estudio anatomo-clínico. *Med Cutan Iber Lat Am* 2: 23–32, 1980.
24. Vicente A, González-Enseñat MA et al. Neonatal erythroderma as a first manifestation of Menkes' disease. *Pediatrics* 130: 239–242, 2012.
25. Kaler SG. Translational research investigations on AT7A: an important human copper ATPase. *Ann NY Acad Sci* 1314: 64–68, 2014.
26. Wee NK, Weinstein DC, Fraser ST et al. The mammalian copper transporters CTR1 and CTR2 and their roles in development and disease. *Int J Biochem Cell Biol* 45: 960–963, 2013.
27. Guillén B, Valencia A, Toledo M et al. Las displasias pilosas. *Dermatol CMQ* 10: 115–122, 2012.
28. Magert HJ, Standker L, Kreutzmann P et al. LEKTI, a novel 15-domain type of human serine proteinase inhibitor. *J Biol Chem* 274: 21499–21502, 1999.
29. Wang S, Olt S, Schoefmann N et al. SPINK5 knockdown in organotypic human skin culture as a model system for Netherton syndrome: effect of genetic inhibition of serine proteases kallikrein 5 and kallikrein 7. *Exp Dermatol* 23: 524–526, 2014.
30. Ito M, Ito K, and Hashimoto K. Pathogenesis in trichorrhexis invaginata (bamboo hair). *J Invest Dermatol* 83: 1–6, 1984.
31. De Berker DAR, Paige DG, Ferguson DJP et al. Golf tee hairs in Netherton's disease. *Pediatr Dermatol* 12: 7–11, 1995.
32. Price VH, Odom RB, Ward WH et al. Trichothiodystrophy. *Arch Dermatol* 116: 1375–1384, 1980.
33. Ferrando J, Mir-Bonafé JM, Cepeda-Valdés R et al. Further insights in trichothiodystrophy: a clinical microscopic, and ultrastructural study of 20 cases and literature review. *Int J Trichology* 4: 158–163, 2012.
34. Malvehy J, Ferrando J, Soler J et al. Trichothiodystrophy associated with urological malformation and primary hypercalciuria. *Pediatr Dermatol* 14: 441–445, 1997.
35. Itin PH and Pittelkow MR. Trichothiodystrophy: review of sulfur-deficient brittle hair syndromes and association with the ectodermal dysplasias. *J Am Acad Dermatol* 22: 705–717, 1990.

36. Tolmie JL, Berker D, Dawber R et al. Syndromes associated with trichothiodystrophy. *Clin Dysmorphol* 3: 1–4, 1991.

37. Singh A, Compe E, Le May N et al. TFIH subunit alterations causing xeroderma pigmentosum and trichothiodystrophy specifically disturb several steps during transcription. *Am J Hum Genet* 96: 194–207, 2015.

38. Kralund HH, Ousager L, Jaspers NG et al. Xeroderma pigmentosum: trichothiodystrophy overlay patient with novel *XPD/ERCC2* mutation *Rare Dis* 1:e24932, 2013.

39. Giglia-Mari GL, Miguel C, Theil F et al. Dynamic interaction of TTDA with TFIIH is stabilized by nucleotide excision repair in living cells. *PLOS Biol* 4e156, 2006.

40. Rudnicka L, Rakowska E, Kerzeja M et al. Hair shafts in trichoscopy: clues for diagnosis of hair and scalp diseases. *Dermatol Clin* 31: 695–708, 2013.

41. Zhu WY and Xia MY. Trichonodosis. *Pediatr Dermatol* 10: 392–393, 1993.

42. Trüeb RM. Trichonodosis neurotica and familial trichonodosis. *J Am Acad Dermatol* 31: 1077, 1994.

43. Leonard JM, Gummer CL, and Dawber RPR. Generalized trichorrhexis nodosa. *Br J Dermatol* 103: 85–90, 1980.

44. Ferrando J, Fontarnau R, Bassas S et al. Expresividad clínica y morfológica de la tricorrexis nodosa. *Dermatol Cosmética* 1: 7–9, 1990.

45. Camacho F. Localized trichorrhexis nodosa. *J Am Acad Dermatol* 20: 696–697, 1989.

46. Pollitt RJ, Jenner FA, and Davies M. Sibs with mental and physical retardation and trichorrhexis nodosa with abnormal amino acid composition of the hair. *Arch Dis Child* 43: 211–216, 1968.

47. Fichtel JC, Richards JA, and Davis LS. Trichorrhexis nodosa secondary to argininosuccinicaciduria. *Pediatr Dermatol* 24: 25–27, 2007.

48. Goulet O, Vinson C, Roquelaure B et al. Syndromic (phenotypic) diarrhea in early infancy. *Orphanet J Rare Dis* 28: 3–6, 2008.

49. Brown VM, Crounse RG, and Abele DC. An unusual new hair shaft abnormality: "bubble hair." *J Am Acad Dermatol* 15: 1113–1117, 1986.

50. Detwiler SP, Carson JL, and Woosley JT. Bubble hair case caused by an overheating hair dryer and reproducibility in normal hair with heat. *J Am Acad Dermatol* 30: 54–60, 1994.

51. Ferrando J, Solé T, and Grimalt R. Scanning electron microscopy details in bubble hair. In *Hair Research for the Next Millennium*. Amsterdam: Elsevier, 1996.

52. Price VH and Gummer CL. Loose anagen hair. *J Am Acad Dermatol* 20: 249–256, 1989.

53. Grimalt R, Barbareschi M, and Menni S. Loose anagen hair of childhood: report of a case and review of the literature. *Eur J Dermatol* 2: 570–572, 1992.

54. KRT75 keratin 75 [*Homo sapiens*]. Gene ID 9119, updated November 1, 2010. http://www.ncbi.nlm.nih.gov/gene/9119

55. SHOC2 soc-2 suppressor of clear homolog (*C. elegans*) [*Homo sapiens*]. Gene ID 8036, updated November 8, 2010. http://www.ncbi.nlm.nih.gov/gene/8036

56. Azón-Masoliver A and Ferrando J. Loose anagen hair in hypohidrotic ectodermal dysplasia. *Pediatr Dermatol* 13: 29–32, 1996.

57. Lo FS, Wang CJ, Wong MC, and Lee NC. Moyamoya disease in two patients with Noonan-like syndrome with loose anagen hair. *Am J Med Genet*, April 9, 2015. doi: 10.1002/ajmg.a.37053.

58. Green J, Fitzpatrick E, de Berker D et al. A gene for pili annulati maps to the telomeric region of chromosome 12q. *J Invest Derm* 123: 1070–1072, 2004.

59. Ferrando J, Fontarnau R, and Hausmann G. Pili annulati. Estudio ultrastructural. *Dermatol Cosmética* 1: 10–11, 1990.

60. Lalevié-Basié B and Polié DJ. Pili annulati. Etude en microscope électronique à balayage. *Ann Dermatol Venereol* 115: 433–440. 1988.

61. Price VH, Thomas RS, and Jones FT. Pseudopili annulati: an unusual variant of normal hair. *Arch Derm* 102: 354–358, 1970.

62. Lee SS, Lee YS, and Giam YC. Pseudopili annulati in a dark-haired individual: a light and electron microscopic study. *Pediatr Derm* 18: 27–30, 2001.

63. Ferrando J, Gratacós R, and Fontarnau R. Woolly hair. Estudio histológico y ultraestructural en cuatro casos. *Actas Dermosifiliogr* 70: 203–214, 1979.

64. Taylor AEM. Hereditary woolly hair with ocular involvement. *Br J Dermatol* 123: 523–525, 1990.

65. Shimomura Y, Wajid M, Petukhova L et al. Autosomal-dominant woolly hair resulting from disruption of keratin 74 (KRT74), a potential determinant of human hair texture. *Am J Hum Genet* 86: 632–638, 2010.

66. Shimomura Y, Wajid M, Ishii Y et al. Disruption of P2RY5, an orphan G protein-coupled receptor, underlies autosomal recessive woolly hair. *Nat Genet* 40: 335–339, 2008.

67. McCoy G, Protonotarios N, Crosby A et al. Identification of a deletion in plakoglobin in arrhythmogenic right ventricular cardiomyopathy with palmoplantar keratoderma and woolly hair (Naxos disease). *Lancet* 355: 2119–2124, 2000.

68. Lantis SDH and Pepper MC. Woolly hair nevus: two case reports and discussion of unruly hair forms. *Arch Dermatol* 114: 233–238, 1978.

69. Peteiro C, Oliva NP, and Zulaica A. Woolly hair nevus: report of a case associated with a verrocous epidermal nevus in the same area. *Pediatr Dermatol* 6: 188–190, 1989.

70. Soler-Carrillo J, Azón-Masoliver A, Malvehy J et al. Nevus de cabello lanoso asociado a alopecia triangular congénita. *Actas Dermosifiliogr* 86: 89–95, 1995.

71. Cullen ST and Fulghum DD. Acquired progressive kinking of the hair. *Arch Dermatol* 125: 252–255, 1989.

72. Ferrando J, Salas J, Vicente A et al. Ensortijamiento adquirido y progresivo del cabello: una forma adquirida de cabello lanoso. *Actas Dermosifiliogr* 84: 235–240, 1993.

73. Rebora A, Chiappara GM, Guarrera M et al. Cheveux crépus acquis un cas fémenin avec revue de la litérature. *Ann Dermatol Venerol* 117: 29–31, 1990.

74. Ormerod AD, Main RA, Ryder ML et al. A family with diffuse partial woolly hair. *Br J Dermatol* 116: 401–405, 1987.

75. Guidetti MS, Fanti BM, Piraccini M et al. Diffuse partial woolly hair. *Acta Derm Venereol* 75: 141–142, 1995.

76. Ferrando J and Grimalt R. Acquired partial curly hair. *Eur J Dermatol* 9: 544–547, 1999.

77. Gibbs RC and Berger RA. Straight-hair nevus. *Int J Dermatol* 9: 47–50, 1970.

78. Day TL. Straight-hair nevus, icththyosis hystrix. *Arch Dermatol* 96: 606, 1967.

79. Lange Wantzin G, Poulsen T, and Thomsen K. Straight-hair nevus in a patient with straight hair. *Acta Dermatol Venereol* 63: 570–571, 1983.

80. Dupré A, Bonafé JL, Litoux F et al. Le syndrome des cheveux incoiffables: pili trianguli et canaliculi. *Ann Dermatol Venerol* 105: 627–630, 1978.

81. Mallon E, Dawber RPR, De Berker D et al. Cheveux incoiffables. Diagnostic, clinical and hair microscopic findings, and pathogenic studies. *Br J Dermatol* 131: 608–614, 1994.

82. Ferrándiz C, Henkes J, Peyrí J et al. Pili canaliculi familiar. *Actas Dermosifiliogr* 71: 225–228, 1980.

83. Salinas CF and Montes GM. Rapp-Hodgkin syndrome: observations on ten cases and characteristic hair changes (pili canaliculi). *Birth Defects Orig Art Ser* 24: 149–168, 1988.

84. Ferrando J, Gratacós MR, Fontarnau R et al. Síndrome de los cabellos impeinables. *Med Cutan Iber Lat Am* 5: 39–46, 1977.

85. Ferrando J, Fontarnau R, Gratacós R et al. Pili canaliculi ("Cheveux incoiffables" ou "Cheveux en fibre de verre"). Dix nouveaux cas avec étude au microscope électronique á balayage. *Ann Dermatol Venerol* 107: 243–248, 1980.

2

Atrichias and Hypotrichoses

Introduction

Most of the clinical and microscopic characteristics of congenital and hereditary hair shaft abnormalities were well described many years ago. Because of this and because many of these conditions have obvious pedigrees, the targeted topical selective gene therapy being developed for hair follicle faults is feasible. Impressive progress has been made in our knowledge of genes that control normal development and anomalies and the search is on to define these genes in hair diseases.

It is not the purpose of this chapter to cover all hypotrichotic syndromes. We cover most of those that have been classified and reviewed the literature to select others that require their undescribed aspects to be explored further.

Congenital Atrichia and Hypotrichosis

Atrichia congenita is characterized by follicular agenesis or programmed follicular destruction. A child may be born with complete absence of scalp and body hair or may progress to that stage in the first 5 years of life. In another variant of the disease, a neonate is born with lanugo hair, which is shed in the first few months of life and never replaced. Caution should be exercised to ensure that a hair abnormality is isolated because other associations may be unveiled only over time.

Congenital hypotrichosis is a less severe form of atrichia congenital; hair is diffusely thinned but not absent. This form usually occurs as an isolated defect. Hypotrichosis may not be noticed until the age of 2 years because of variations in the quality and quantity of hair normally present at birth.

Most cases of congenital hypotrichosis and atrichia congenita are autosomal recessive (AR) traits. Several autosomal dominant (AD) pedigrees have been identified. When no family history is obtained, a scalp biopsy should be performed to exclude alopecia areata totalis. A biopsy will also provide information about follicle architecture and count and reveals other cutaneous abnormalities.

The conditions that present with hypotrichosis without complete alopecia in infancy constitute a very long list. The hypotrichosis may be secondary to follicular hypoplasia or to faulty hair shaft production and breakage. Many of the ectodermal dysplasias are associated with hypotrichosis, but unfortunately most hair shaft abnormalities have not been well characterized. Abnormal hair is generally described clinically only as brittle, sparse, or lusterless.

Numerous attempts have been made to classify the conditions characterized by congenital alopecia or hypotrichosis. In 1892, Bonnet [1] proposed the first known classification based on embryological principles. It has been widely used until now and roughly divides congenital hypotrichoses with normal ectodermal structures from those with associated teeth and nail defects. Cockayne [2] and Muller [3] later attempted a more critical analysis by proposing a working classification that allowed the currently named syndromes to be identified and provided provisional status for those not yet characterized. After the Berlin Congress in 1981, Sâlamon [4] proposed a classification for the global problem of hair loss that is considered one of the most useful systems for the study of congenital hypotrichosis.

In recent years, major breakthroughs in genomic techniques yielded considerable progress toward unraveling the molecular bases of inherited skin diseases. At present, over 6000 Mendelian disorders

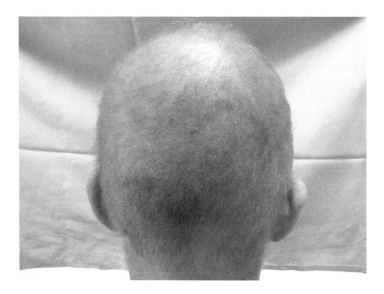

FIGURE 2.1   Many congenital hypotrichoses not associated with other defects cannot be classified properly.

are known; 560 involve skin abnormalities and are associated with more than 500 unique protein-coding genes. More than 300 inherited disorders featuring hair abnormalities have been catalogued to date, and yet no genetic defects have been identified in a substantial number of the disorders (Figures 2.1 and 2.2) [5].

This new knowledge led to a reorganization of the classification systems for this group of diseases. Instead of being based solely on clinical findings, the classification now integrates both clinical and molecular features. It is now possible to assign most forms of hypotrichosis to one gene (or group of genes) on the basis of limited information about three clinical features: mode of inheritance, presence or absence of associated features, and microscopic appearance of hair shafts. When such data are available, it is easy to decide the optimal molecular diagnostic strategy and order genetic testing that is likely to lead to a correct diagnosis (Table 2.1). As Betz et al. [5] indicate, most patients with hypotrichoses can be assigned to a group of molecularly defined hair disorders using three clinical criteria.

In this review, we will follow the practical classification based on the clinical observations proposed

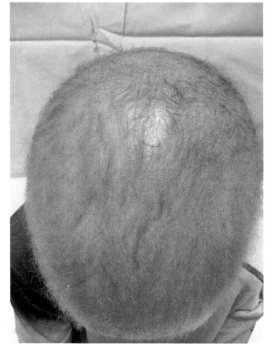

FIGURE 2.2   In non-classified congenital hypotrichosis, no hair shaft alterations are present.

by Camacho [6]. Readers should be aware, however, that each group covers a large clinical spectrum of disorders that are not grouped on a pathogenetic basis. The classification scheme in Table 2.2 is largely of didactic value.

TABLE 2.1

Clinicogenetic Classification of Hypotrichoses

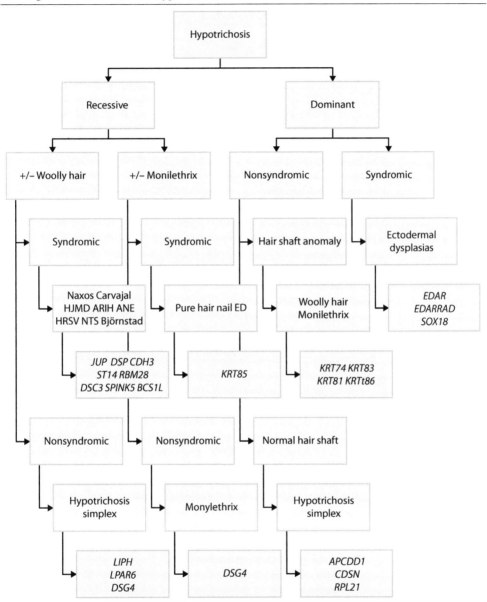

Source: Adapted from Betz RC et al. *J Invest Dermatol* 132: 906–914, 2012.

Note: Using three clinical criteria, most patients with hypotrichosis can be assigned to a group of molecularly defined hair disorders. ANE: Alopecia, neurological defects, and endocrinopathy; ARIH: Autosomal recessive ichthyosis with hypotrichosis; DSG4: Desmoglein 4; ED: Ectodermal dysplasia; EDAR: Ectodysplasin A receptor; EDARADD: EDAR-associated death domain; HJMD: Hypotrichosis with juvenile macular dystrophy; HRSV: Hypotrichosis with recurrent vesicles; KRT85: Keratin 85; LIPH: Lipase H; LPAR6: Lysophosphatidic acid receptor 6; NTS: Netherton syndrome.

TABLE 2.2

Classification of Generalized Congenital and Hereditary Alopecias

1. Genodermatoses with non-scarring hypotrichosis
   1.1 With skeletal alterations
        McKusich disease or chondrodysplasia
        Moynahan disease (hypotrichosis, syndactyly, retinitis)
        Trichorhinophalangeal syndromes
        Pierre-Robin syndrome
        Cardio-facial cutaneous syndrome
        Alopecia-contracture-dwarfism (ACD) syndrome with mental retardation
        Oculo-dental-digital syndrome
        Dubowitz syndrome
        Noonan syndrome
        Hallemann-Streiff syndrome
   1.2 With ectodermic alterations
        Ectodermal dysplasias
   1.3 With neuroectodermal alterations
        Tricothiodystrophy
   1.4 With chromosomal alterations
        Down syndrome
        Klinefelter syndrome
        Turner syndrome
   1.5 With amino acid metabolism alterations
        Hypotrichosis, hair shaft defect, hypercysteine hair, and glucosuria syndrome
        Citrulinemia
        Hartnup disease
        Homocystinuria
        Phenylketonuria
        Tyrosinemias I and II
   1.6 Other genodermatoses with hypotrichosis
        1.6.1 Progerias
               Werner syndrome or pangeria
               Hutchinson-Gilford syndrome or childhood progeria
               Variot-Cailleau syndrome or childhood gerodermia
               Other progerias
        1.6.2 Others
               Congenital ichthyosiform erythrodermia
               Netherton syndrome
               Tay syndrome
               Rud syndrome
               KID syndrome
               Rothmund-Thomson disease
               Poikilodermia–alopecia–retrognathism–cleft palate syndrome
               Zinsser-Cole-Engman disease
               Kallin syndrome or epidermolysis bullosa simplex
   1.7 Genodermatoses with hypotrichosis and tumors
        Rombo syndrome
        Bazex-Dupré-Christol syndrome
   1.8 Hereditary simple hypotrichosis

Continued

TABLE 2.2 (Continued)

Classification of Generalized Congenital and Hereditary Alopecias

2. Genodermatoses with scarring hypotrichosis
2.1 Darier disease
2.2 Ichthyosis X
2.3 Dystrophic epidermolysis bullosa
2.4 Incontinentia pigmenti
2.5 Polyostotic fibrous dysplasia
2.6 Conradi syndrome
2.7 Happle syndrome

Generalized Congenital Alopecia

Genodermatoses with Non-Scarring Hypotrichosis

Genodermatoses with Skeletal Alterations

Trichorhinophalangeal Syndromes

Trichorhinophalangeal syndromes (TRPSs) constitute distinctive combinations of hair, facial, and bone abnormalities with AD inheritance. Three types are described below.

Trichorhinophalangeal syndrome type I is characterized clinically by a variable congenital hypotrichosis, piriform (pear-shaped) nose, coniform epiphysis, subnasal fold, thin lips, prognatia, and mandibular hypoplasia (Figure 2.3). The hair alterations consist of diffuse alopecia with a broad forehead and partial alopecia of the lateral third of the eyebrows. Scanning electron microscopic studies of hair shafts can reveal flattened hairs with an elliptoid transverse section pattern. Mechanical behavior of the hair may be abnormal and reveal a significant increase in the viscous parameter indicating decreased intermolecular bridging within the keratin matrix [7].

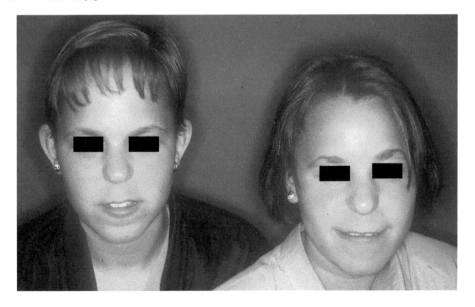

FIGURE 2.3   In trichorhinophalangeal syndrome, the face displays characteristic dwarfism, diffuse hypotrichosis, piriform nose, and elongated philtrum.

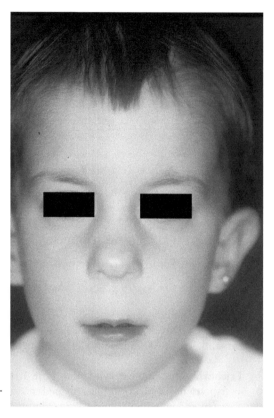

FIGURE 2.4   Typical facies of trichorhinophalangeal syndrome with piriform nose.

Trichorhinophalangeal syndrome type II (Langer-Giedion syndrome). Patients with type II usually present with hypotrichosis of the scalp hair, piriform nose, and redundant skin as in type I along with multiple cartilaginous exostoses. Lu et al. [8] described alterations to this syndrome including aplasia of the epiglottis and congenital nephrotic syndrome.

Trichorhinophalangeal syndrome type III is a newly defined clinical entity [9] inherited as an AD trait and clinically characterized by growth retardation, craniofacial abnormalities, severe brachydactyly, and sparse hair. The absence of mental retardation and cartilaginous exostoses is required for the diagnosis of type III. Other associated abnormalities include short stature, a thin upper lip and prominent lower lip, a pear-shaped nose, stubby fingers and toes with cone-shaped epiphyses, and sparse scalp hair (Figures 2.4 through 2.6).

Dubowitz Syndrome

First described in 1965, Dubowitz syndrome (DS) is characterized by a peculiar face, eczema, small stature, and mild microcephaly. The cutaneous findings consist of eczematous eruptions affecting the face and flexural areas [10]. Scalp hair is sparse and brittle and commonly affects the lateral eyebrows. Patients affected by DS have moderate mental deficiencies with a tendency toward hyperactivity, short attention spans, stubbornness, and shyness and have been characterized by their high-pitched weak cries.

Hallermann-Streiff Syndrome

Hallermann-Streiff syndrome is a rare congenital anomaly characterized by a peculiar bird face, mandibular and maxillary hypoplasias, dyscephaly, congenital cataracts, microphthalmia, hypotrichosis, skin atrophy, and short stature [11]. Dental abnormalities are present in 80% of cases and include malocclusion, crowding, severe caries, supernumerary and neonatal teeth, enamel hypoplasia, hypodontia, premature eruption of primary dentition, agenesis of permanent teeth, and anterior displacement or absence of condyles [12].

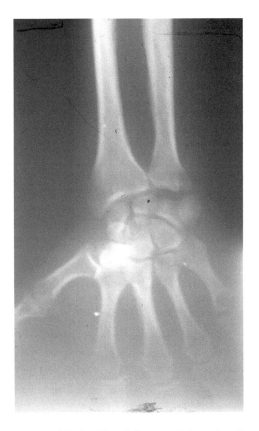

FIGURE 2.5   Radiography reveals cone epiphysis of first phalanges and shortening of some metatarsi.

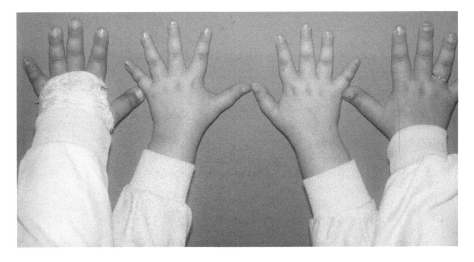

FIGURE 2.6   Clinical observation of hands showing shortening of metatarsi.

Genodermatoses with Ectodermal Alterations

Ectodermal Dysplasias

Ectodermal dysplasias (EDs) are a heterogeneous group of conditions primarily affecting the hair, teeth, nails, and skin, and are classified according to the tissues affected. EDs are rare diseases with an estimated incidence of only 7 in 10,000 births [13]. Of the 170 EDs described to date, fewer than 30 have been explained at the molecular level via identification of the causative genes.

The ectodermal dysplasia term was originally applied to anhidrotic ectodermal dysplasia in which hair, teeth, nails, and sweat glands are defective. The classification proposed by Freire-Maia in 1977 [14] was based on a primary defect of ectodermal derivatives. Conditions in which the ectodermal changes are secondary as in xeroderma pigmentosum are thus excluded from the EDs. According to Freire-Maia's classifications, subgroup 1 is hair dysplasia; subgroup 2, dental dysplasia; subgroup 3, nail dysplasia; subgroup 4, sweat gland defects; and subgroup 5, defects of other ectodermal structures. In 1980, Solomon and Keuer [15] defined ED subgroups based on the ectodermal structures affected (Table 2.3).

Anhidrotic Ectodermal Dysplasia (Christ-Touraine Syndrome)

In this X-linked syndrome, sweat glands and other ectodermal-derived appendages are absent or few in number. The full syndrome occurs only in males. Scalp and body hair is short, fine, and very sparse and often brightly colored; it may increase in quantity after puberty. Eyebrows and eyelashes may also be sparse or absent but may be minimally affected. The prominent square forehead, saddle nose, thick lower

TABLE 2.3

Ectodermal Dysplasia Subgroups Proposed by Solomon and Keuer

Subgroups 1, 2, 3, and 4 (hair, teeth, nails, and sweating defects)
    Anhidrotic ectodermal dysplasia
    Rapp-Hodgkin
    Ectrodactyly–ectodermal dysplasia–cleft palate syndrome
    Popliteal web syndrome
    Xeroderma–talipes–enamel defect syndrome
Subgroups 1, 2, and 3 (hair, teeth, and nail defects)
    Clouston dysplasia
    Trichodento-osseous syndrome
    Ellis-van Creveld syndrome
    Ankyloblepharon–ectodermal defect–cleft palate syndrome
    Basan syndrome
    Tooth–nail syndrome
Subgroups 1, 3, and 4 (hair, nails, and sweating defects)
    Freire-Maia syndrome
Subgroups 1 and 2 (hair and teeth defects)
    Orofaciodigital syndrome I
    Sensenbrenner syndrome
    Trichodental syndrome
Subgroups 1 and 3 (hair and nail defects)
    Curly hair–ankyloblepharon–nail dysplasia syndrome
    Onychotrichodysplasia with neutropenia
Subgroup 1 (hair defects)
    Trichorhinophalangeal syndromes
    Dubowitz syndrome
    Moynahan syndrome

Source: Solomon LM and Keuer EJ. The ectodermal dysplasias. *Arch Dermatol* 116: 1295–1299, 1980. With permission.

lip, and pointed chin produce a distinctive face. The skin around the eyes is finely wrinkled and may be pigmented. The teeth may be absent or few in number, and the canines and incisors are characteristically cone shaped.

Absent or reduced sweating leads to heat intolerance, and unexplained pyrexia may be the presenting symptom in infancy. Carrier females may be clinically normal but may show one or more of the features of the syndrome such as conical teeth, hypotrichosis, or heat intolerance. Otherwise apparently normal carriers may show dermatoglyphic abnormalities, the presence of which may aid diagnosis [16]. See Figures 2.7 and 2.8.

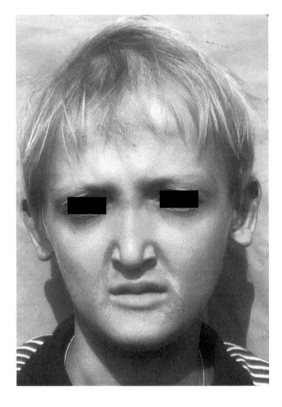

FIGURE 2.7 Typical facies of anhidrotic ectodermal dysplasia.

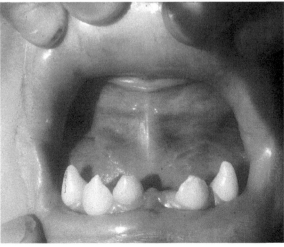

FIGURE 2.8 Conical incisors in a male affected by hypohidrotic ectodermal dysplasia.

Ectrodactyly, Ectodermal Dysplasia, and Cleft Lip and Palate (EEC Syndrome)

The association of ectrodactyly (lobster-claw deformity), ectodermal dysplasia, and cleft lip and palate is a well-defined AD syndrome [16]. Reported EEC syndrome cases show sparse hair, malformed teeth with early caries, ectrodactyly, cleft lip and/or palate, lacrimal duct stenosis, and kidney abnormalities, but not all defects are present in all affected individuals within a single family.

Hypotrichosis with Juvenile Macular Dystrophy (HJMD)

Becker et al. [17] described two sisters in a family of consanguineous parents who exhibited diffuse hypotrichosis of the head and visual impairment in the context of a tricho-ocular malformation of an ectodermal dysplasia. This entity is an AR disorder. Mutations in the *P-cadherin* (*CDH3*) gene have been shown to underlie HJMD. Because *P-cadherin* is expressed in the hair follicles and also in the retinal pigmented epithelium of the eye, its disruption would lead to macular dystrophy of the retina [18].

Hypotrichoses with Amino Acid Metabolism Alteration and Ectodermal Dysplasia

Hypotrichosis, Hair-Shaft Structure Defects, Hypercysteine Hair, and Glucosuria

Blume-Peytavi et al. [19] reported two Turkish siblings with fragile and sparse scalp hair associated with glucosuria without diabetes or kidney disease. Clinical examination revealed normal physical and mental development, and an analysis of plucked hairs showed dysplastic and broken hair shafts. Polarizing microscopy and scanning electron microscopic studies revealed torsion, irregularities, and impressions of the hair shaft as seen in *pili torti*, trichorrhexis nodosa, and pseudomonilethrix. Analysis of the amino acid composition of the hair demonstrated a significant reduction of sulfonic cysteic acid and elevated cysteine and lanthionine contents (Figures 2.9 through 2.12).

Other Genodermatoses with Hypotrichosis

Keratitis, Ichthyosis, and Deafness (KID) Syndrome

KID syndrome is a congenital ectodermal disorder that affects the epidermis and other ectodermal-derived tissues such as the corneal epithelium and the inner ear. In a classic review [20], 61 patients who met the criteria for this syndrome were identified. All had cutaneous and auditory abnormalities, and 95% also revealed ophthalmologic defects. The most frequent clinical features were neurosensory deafness (90%), erythrokeratoderma (89%), vascularizing keratitis (79%), alopecia (79%), and reticulated hyperkeratosis of the palms and soles (41%).

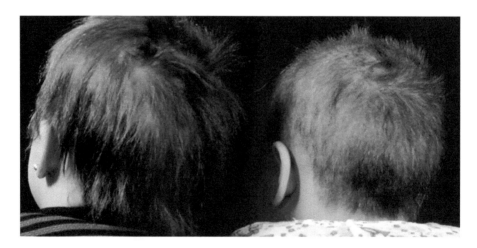

FIGURE 2.9   Siblings with hypotrichosis, hair shaft structure defects, hypercysteine hair, and glucosuria. (Courtesy of Professor U. Blume-Peytavi.)

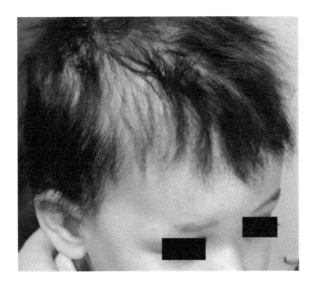

FIGURE 2.10   Detail of one sibling with sparse and fragile hair. (Courtesy of Professor U. Blume-Peytavi.)

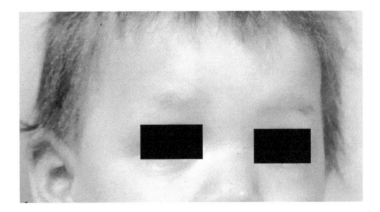

FIGURE 2.11   Eyebrows and eyelashes were also affected. (Courtesy of Professor U. Blume-Peytavi.)

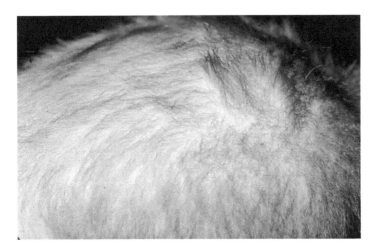

FIGURE 2.12   Detail of posterior part of scalp demonstrating short and fragile hair. (Courtesy of Professor U. Blume-Peytavi.)

In the same article, the authors stated that the KID acronym does not accurately define this entity. The disorder is not an ichthyosis because scaling is not the main cutaneous feature. In addition, not all patients have keratitis. They suggest that this syndrome should be included under the general heading of congenital ectodermal defects as a keratodermatous ectodermal dysplasia (KED); see Figures 2.13 through 2.15.

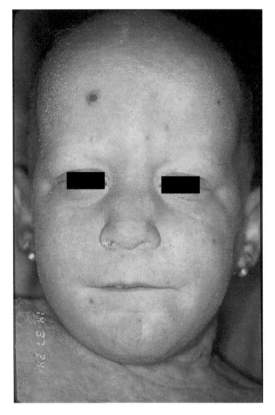

FIGURE 2.13   KID syndrome. Typical facies with hypotrichosis.

FIGURE 2.14   Detail of spiny ichthyosis.

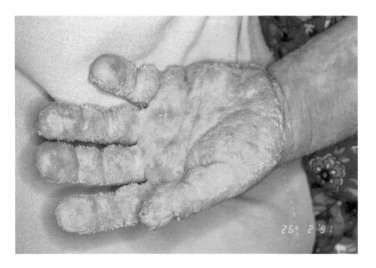

FIGURE 2.15   Spiny palmar keratoderma.

Genodermatoses with Hypotrichosis and Tumors

Rombo Syndrome

First described by Michaëlsson in 1981 [21], Rombo syndrome is an AD disease clinically characterized by hypotrichosis affecting the eyelashes and yellowish follicular facial papules. Patients also present with cyanotic lips and multiple tricoepitheliomata and basal cell carcinomas [22].

Bazex-Dupré-Christol Syndrome

Bazex-Dupré-Christol syndrome (BDCS) is an X-linked dominant disorder of the hair follicles characterized by follicular atrophoderma, multiple basal cell carcinomas, hypotrichosis, milia, and localized hypohidrosis [23]. Follicular atrophodermas (FAs) are follicular depressions ("ice pick marks") seen commonly on the dorsa of the hands and elbows.

Kidd et al. [24] described five affected members with this syndrome through three generations of a Scottish family. The reported patients showed hypohidrosis confined to the face, coarse hair, dry skin, milia, and follicular atrophoderma. All the adults had histories of multiple basal cell carcinomas. None of them presented skeletal features suggestive of Gorlin syndrome. The authors thus suggest that BDCS should be considered as a differential diagnosis in patients with early onset or familial basal cell carcinomas.

In 1994 Goeteyn et al. [25] described 20 affected patients of a large family across four generations with typical features of BDCS. However, the clinical picture within the family differed with regard to gender and age, confirming an X-linked inheritance; see Figures 2.16 and 2.17.

Hereditary Hypotrichosis Simplex

Hereditary hypotrichosis simplex (HHS) is an uncommon group of familial hypotrichias and atrichias, usually non-scarring, and not associated with other dysplasias or internal abnormalities. HHS is an AD hair disorder characterized by progressive loss of hair starting in the middle of the first decade of life [18,26]. HHS can be largely classified as the scalp-limited form (HHSS) [27] and the generalized form (GHHS) in which facial and body hairs are also affected.

HHSS was previously mapped to chromosome 6p21. Heterozygous nonsense mutations in the *CDSN* gene were identified later in patients with HHSS. Interestingly, it has been shown that homozygous mutations in the *CDSN* gene underlie an inflammatory type of generalized peeling skin syndrome characterized by erythema with peeling of the cornified layer over the whole body.

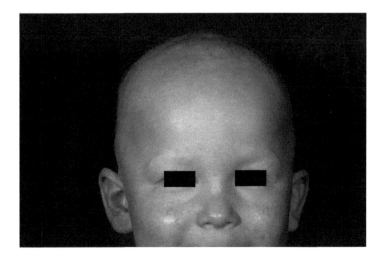

FIGURE 2.16   Bazex-Dupré-Christol syndrome. Typical facies of 4-year-old boy with scalp hypotrichosis and fine, light blonde, irregularly curly hair. (Courtesy of Professor M.L. Geerts.)

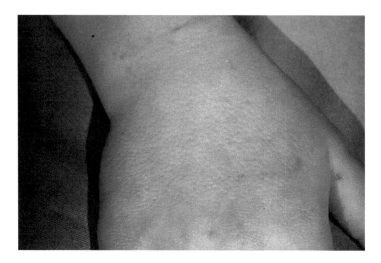

FIGURE 2.17   Typical depressions on dorsa of hands (follicular atrophoderma).

It is also known that mutations in other genes functionally related to *CDSN* can show some hair phenotypes. Of these, Netherton syndrome is an AR disorder characterized by ichthyosiform erythroderma, atopic manifestations, and a hair shaft anomaly called bamboo hair (trichorrhexis invaginata). Netherton syndrome is caused by mutations in the *SPINK5* gene. More recent reports indicate that recessively inherited mutations in the *ST14* gene underlie ichthyosis with hypotrichosis syndrome [18].

The generalized form of HHS (GHHS) was previously mapped to chromosome 18p11.32–11.23. Recently, a heterozygous mutation in the *APCDD1* gene was identified in families with GHHS.

Recently Described Syndromes (Non-Classified Disorders)

In the past decade, several hypotrichotic syndromes have been described as new genodermatoses or new syndromes. They have yet to be classified and included into the older classification schemes.

Congenital Ichthyosis with Follicular Atrophoderma

Lestringant et al. [28] described five Emirati siblings (three girls and two boys), aged 4 to 18 years old, with normal stature, diffuse congenital ichthyosis, patchy follicular atrophoderma, generalized and diffuse non-scarring hypotrichosis, and marked hypohidrosis. Steroid sulfatase activity, assessed in the two boys, was found normal. Electron microscopic studies of ichthyotic skin did not show specific abnormalities. The patients were thought to have Bazex syndrome; however, ichthyosis is not a component of the syndrome. The authors concluded that congenital ichthyosis with follicular atrophoderma represents a new AR genodermatosis (Figures 2.18 and 2.19).

Congenital Atrichia, Palmoplantar Hyperkeratosis, Mental Retardation, and Early Loss of Teeth

Steijlen et al. [29] reported four siblings with congenital atrichia, palmoplantar hyperkeratosis, mental retardation, and early loss of teeth. The pedigree of the family suggested an AR trait. This combination of findings was not reported previously and is therefore considered a new genetic entity.

Keratoderma, Hypotrichosis, and Leukonychia Totalis

Basaran et al. [30] reported three relatives with congenital hypotrichosis characterized by trichorrhexis nodosa and trichoptilosis, dry skin, keratosis pilaris, and leukonychia totalis. The patients also developed a progressive transgrediens type of palmoplantar keratoderma and hyperkeratotic lesions on the knees, elbows, and perianal region.

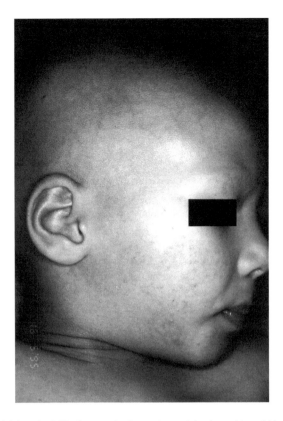

FIGURE 2.18 Congenital ichthyosis, follicular atrophoderma, hypotrichosis, and hypohidrosis (Lestringant syndrome). Clinical aspects of facies of patient. (Courtesy of Dr. G.G. Lestringant.)

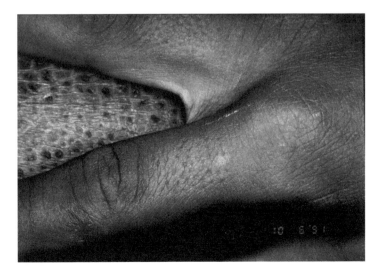

FIGURE 2.19 Follicular atrophoderma and ichthyosis.

Alopecia–Mental Retardation Syndrome Associated with Convulsions and Hypergonadotropic Hypogonadism

Devriendt et al. [31] reported two brothers with total congenital alopecia, mental retardation, childhood convulsions, and hypergonadotropic hypogonadism. The authors believe that this association that was not reported previously represents a new AR condition.

Universal Congenital Alopecia

Complete or partial congenital absence of hair may occur in isolation or with associated abnormalities. Most families with isolated congenital alopecia have been reported to follow an AR inheritance. In an attempt to map the gene for the AR form, Nothem et al. [32] performed genetic linkage analysis of a large inbred family from Pakistan whose affected members showed complete absence of hair. The authors mapped the gene for this hereditary form of isolated congenital alopecia on chromosome 8p21–22 and named it alopecia universalis congenitalis (ALUNC). In a later article [33], they reported a homozygous missense mutation in the hairless (*HR*) gene. They also found that the *human hairless* gene undergoes alternative splicing and that at least two isoforms generated by alternative usage of exon 17 are found in human tissues.

Interestingly, the isoform containing exon 17 is the predominant isoform expressed in all tissues except the skin (where the authors observed exclusive expression of the shorter isoform). They speculate that this tissue-specific difference in the proportion of hairless transcripts lacking exon 17 sequences may contribute to the tissue-specific disease phenotype observed in individuals with this type of isolated congenital alopecia.

Atrichia with Papular Lesions

Atrichia with papular lesions (APL) is a rare AR disorder characterized by early onset of complete hair loss followed by papular eruptions due to formation of dermal cysts. It has been shown that loss-of-function mutations in the *HR* gene underlie APL [18]. It has been reported in patients with congenital hypotrichosis and milia. These patients presented with coarse, sparse hair and multiple milia on the face, chest, axillae, and pubic region. No abnormalities of teeth and nails were found. Polarizing light microscopy of hair showed increased diameters of hair shafts. Rapelanoro et al. [34] reported a large four-generation family whose members presented with congenital hypotrichosis and multiple self-healing milia.

Marie Unna Hereditary Hypotrichosis

Typical patients are born with normal to adequate or normal to coarse hair. With increasing age, the hair becomes increasingly coarse and wiry, and has been likened to an ill-fitting wig or a horse's mane. Patients commonly have minimal or absent eyebrows, eyelashes, and body hair, including secondary sexual hair. They often demonstrate a progressive, non-scarring loss of scalp hair that begins around puberty, particularly in the vertex and scalp margins. The eventual result may be only a sparse fringe of remaining hair along the scalp periphery [35].

Marie Unna hereditary hypotrichosis has only rarely been associated with coexisting abnormalities. Specifically, up to 50% of affected individuals may demonstrate exceptionally widely spaced upper incisor teeth. Additionally, reports have been made of associations with Ehlers-Danlos syndrome and juvenile macular examination; gentle hair pulling may extract multiple anagen hairs. Light microscopic examination may reveal hair shafts that are deeply pigmented and vary in diameter. Hairs may also be twisted or bent at odd angles. Histologic findings include a significantly reduced number of follicles per unit area that are often atrophic. A mild to moderate inflammatory infiltrate with limited fibrosis and scarring may be present.

Marie Unna hypotrichosis was mapped to chromosome 8p21.3, where the *HR* gene is located. It is related to upregulation of the expression of this gene [18]; see Figures 2.20 through 2.24.

Genodermatoses with Scarring Alopecia

Happle Syndrome

Gobello et al. [36] described a 13-year-old girl with chondrodysplasia punctata associated with ichthyosis arranged along Blaschko's lines, follicular atrophoderma, cicatricial alopecia, and coarse lusterless

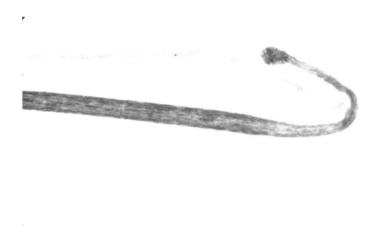

FIGURE 2.20   Dystrophic hair shaft and root in patient affected by Marie Unna hypotrichosis.

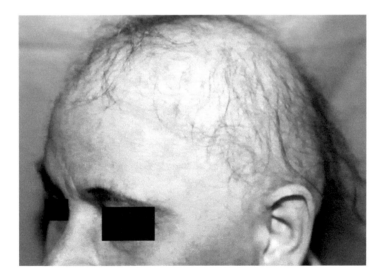

FIGURE 2.21   Patient with typical aspect of Marie Unna hypotrichosis. (Courtesy of Professor F.M. Camacho.)

hair. The patient also showed a congenital cataract in the right eye, dysplastic facial appearance, and symmetrical shortening of the tubular bones. The pathogenetic concept of functional X-chromosome mosaicism introduced by Happle is the source of the name of this syndrome.

Localized Congenital Alopecias

Congenital Triangular Alopecia

Congenital triangular alopecia (CTA), also known as temporal triangular alopecia [37], is a unilateral or less frequent bilateral patch of non-cicatricial and non-inflammatory alopecia in the frontotemporal region. Although CTA is a congenital trait, it is usually noticed when a child is more than 2 years of age. Only about 74 cases have been reported [38], probably because the lesions are benign and non-progressive. An estimated frequency of 0.11% was reported by García-Hernández et al. [39].

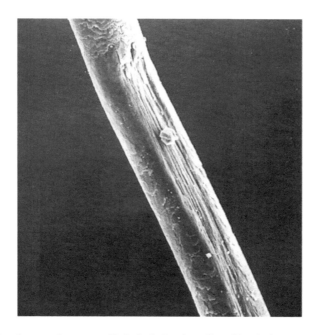

FIGURE 2.22   Scanning electron microscopy of hair shaft of patient affected by Marie Unna hypotrichosis.

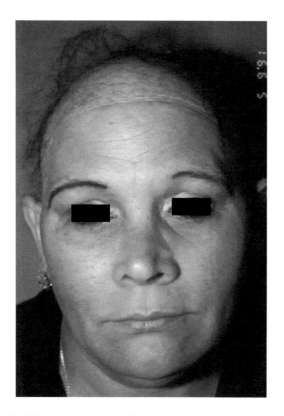

FIGURE 2.23   Patient with Marie Unna hypotrichosis without wig. (Courtesy of Professor F.M. Camacho.)

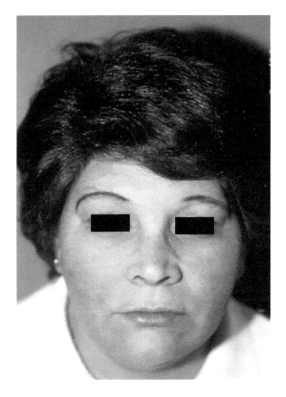

FIGURE 2.24   Same patient with wig. (Courtesy of Professor F.M. Camacho.)

Most cases are sporadic but the trait may affect several members of a family, although this is exceptional. The hair loss is described as a triangular, oval, or lancet-shaped temporal patch covered only by vellus hair. Recently, a central hair tuft in CTA has been described as a typical feature of this disorder in a substantial number of cases [40].

CTA usually occurs as an isolated anomaly but several congenital diseases have been associated with it, for example, phakomatosis pigmentovascularis, Down syndrome, Dandy-Walker malformation, mental retardation, seizures, congenital heart diseases, bone and tooth abnormalities, multiple lentigines, and café-au-lait patches (Figures 2.25 and 2.26).

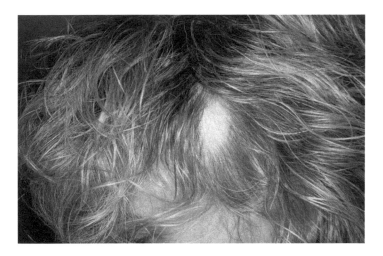

FIGURE 2.25   Congenital triangular alopecia is usually oval shaped.

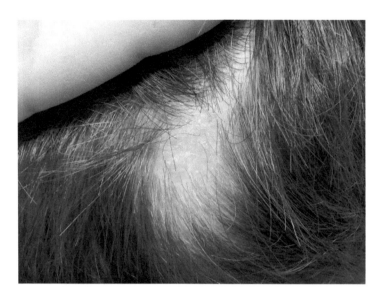

FIGURE 2.26   Differential diagnosis from nevus sebaceous must be performed.

Aplasia Cutis Congenita

Aplasia cutis congenita is one of a heterogeneous group of disorders characterized by the absence of a portion of skin in a localized or widespread area of the scalp at birth. It usually manifests as a solitary defect on the scalp, but may occur as multiple lesions. Aplasia cutis is a congenital condition in which skin, bone, and dura may be absent. Most cases affect the scalp and are limited to the dermis and epidermis. Vertex aplasia cutis typically ranges in size from 0.5 to 3 cm. Ultrasound and magnetic resonance imaging are helpful diagnostic tools for determining the extents of lesions (Figures 2.27 through 2.29).

Adams-Oliver Syndrome

This syndrome depends on the association of aplasia cutis with terminal digital abnormalities, namely, shortening of the fingers and toes, absence of phalanges, or, more rarely, the absence of an entire extremity. A literature review [41] revealed a rate of 13.4% for congenital heart malformations in individuals

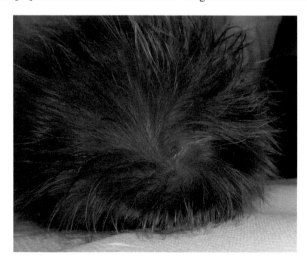

FIGURE 2.27   Aplasia cutis congenita. (Courtesy of Dr. Mario Cutrone.)

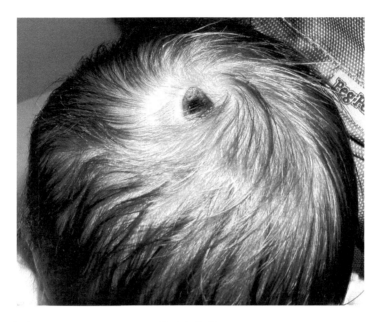

FIGURE 2.28   Aplasia cutis congenita. (Courtesy of Dr. Mario Cutrone.)

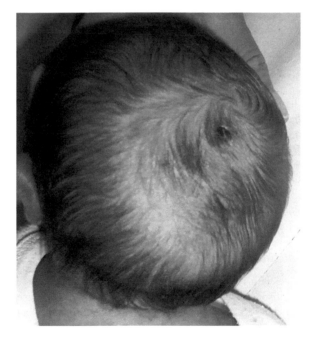

FIGURE 2.29   Aplasia cutis congenita. (Courtesy of Dr. Mario Cutrone.)

with Adams-Oliver syndrome, suggesting that cardiac anomalies are frequent manifestations. Thus, all patients with Adams-Oliver syndrome should be evaluated for cardiac abnormalities.

Aplasia Cutis Congenita and Associated Disorders

Gershoni-Baruch and Leibo [42] reported two siblings with congenital nystagmus, cone–rod dysfunction, high myopia, and aplasia cutis congenita on the midline of the scalp vertex. The authors consider this familial oculocutaneous condition a new and unique AR disorder.

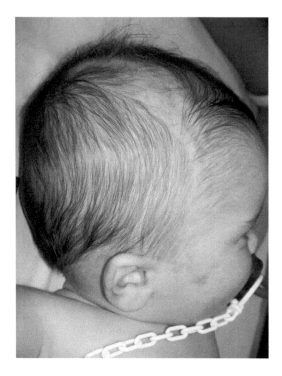

FIGURE 2.30   Nevus sebaceous may be very large. (Courtesy of Dr. Mario Cutrone.)

Nevus Sebaceous of Jadassohn

This benign, congenital hamartoma of the folliculo-sebaceous apocrine unit and epidermis that often presents at birth appears to regress in childhood and grows during puberty, suggesting possible hormonal control. A childhood lesion consists of a linear, round, or irregular circumscribed, hairless, yellow-orange, waxy, pebble-like papule or plaque. In puberty, the lesion becomes verrucous and nodular. Nevus sebaceous patients may develop tumors in adulthood, particularly syringocystadenoma papilliferum and benign hair follicle tumors. Basal cell carcinoma has been observed in about 5% of cases (Figures 2.30 and 2.31)

Other Infrequent Unclassifiable Conditions

Chondrodysplasia Punctata (Conradi-Hünermann Syndrome)

Chondrodysplasia punctata with rhizomelic nanism or Conradi-Hünermann syndrome is the clinical expression of a functional disorder of cellular peroxisomes. It leads to decreased synthesis of plasmalogens with pointed calcium deposits in endochondral tissues (chondrodysplasia punctata) and rhizomelic nanism [43].

The syndrome is accompanied by several little known cutaneous signs. Ichthyosiform eruption is shown during the first months of life. In about 25% of cases, it resolves spontaneously. It has been described as similar to pressed egg shells on an underlying erythematous condition; dyschromia with a spiral disposition similar to that of incontinentia pigmenti, probably related to residual lesions left by the prior ichthyosiform eruption; follicular atrophoderma, probably of the same origin; and cicatricial alopecia in plaques.

Clinical diagnosis: From a dermatological view, a clinician must consider this chondrodysplasia punctata when treating an infant who shows an atypical ichthyosiform eruption (erythroderma with a pressed egg shell appearance) and congenital plaques of cicatricial alopecia. It should

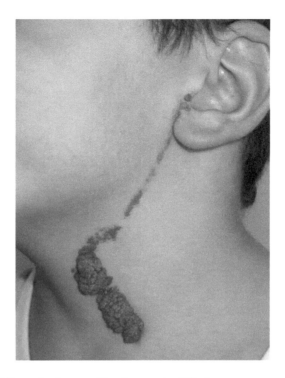

FIGURE 2.31   Differential diagnosis of nevus epidermicus may be difficult.

also be considered for children or youths with rhizomelic nanism, plaques of cicatricial alope-cia, and "swirling" dyschromia and/or follicular atrophoderma. The presence of chondrodys-plasia punctata in the epiphyses of long bones and other locations will confirm the diagnosis.

Histology: The biopsy results from inflammatory lesions of the first phase are compatible with congenital ichthyosiform erythroderma. Biopsies of the alopecic plaques will confirm cicatri-cial alopecia: atrophy with peripilar fibrosis (Figures 3.32 through 2.36).

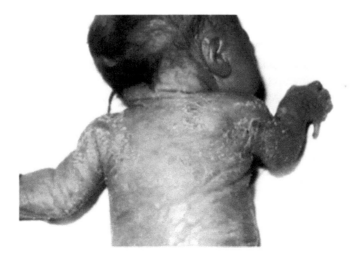

FIGURE 2.32   Skin of patient affected by Conradi-Hünermann syndrome shows eggshell-like ichthyosis. (Courtesy of Dr. González Otero.)

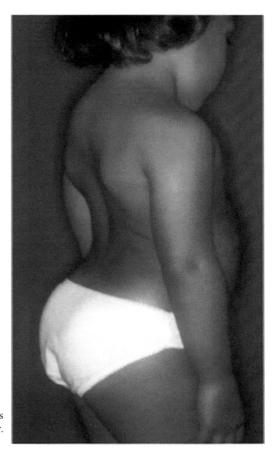

FIGURE 2.33 Skeletal alterations are common in patients affected by Conradi-Hünermann syndrome. (Courtesy of Dr. González Otero.)

Keratosis Follicularis Decalvans (Siemens Syndrome)

This disorder is included along with atrophic facial keratosis follicularis and atrophoderma vermicularis in the follicular keratosis decalvans group. It is usually sporadic but familial cases have been described. It is characteristically a congenital hypotrichosis with pronounced hyperkeratosis follicularis on the scalp (in this sense it is similar to monilethrix), face, and entire body. It especially affects the eyebrows, where intense underlying erythema is observed.

The evolution progresses over time leading to a generalized diffuse alopecia. It may be associated with photophobia, ocular alterations (blepharitis, conjunctivitis, keratitis) caused by ocular and lacrimal dryness, mental retardation, retarded development of height and weight, deafness, microcephaly, ungual hypoplasia, and palmoplantar hyperkeratosis [44]. Its recent association with ductus arteriosus and hypospadias suggests a new syndromic association [45].

> **Histology:** The scalp shows a pattern of diffuse cicatricial alopecia with absence or hypoplasia of the sebaceous glands. Other findings are atrophic hair follicles with fibrosis, atrophic or cicatricial dermic changes, and absence or hypoplasia of sebaceous glands.
>
> **Clinical diagnosis:** Diffuse congenital hypotrichosis of the scalp and eyebrows with pronounced generalized hyperkeratosis follicularis, especially in the hairy areas, is present. The disorder must be differentiated from monilethrix in which the follicular hyperkeratosis is much more pronounced in the occipital region and tends to improve over time. This does not occur in keratosis follicularis.
>
> **Treatment:** The follicular hyperkeratosis improves with retinoids or topical alpha hydroxyl acids.

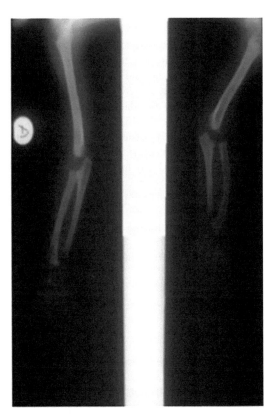

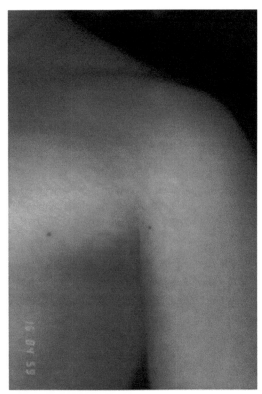

FIGURE 2.34 Limb x-ray reveals chondrodysplasia. (Courtesy of Dr. González Otero.)

FIGURE 2.35 Detail of skin of patient affected by Conradi-Hünermann syndrome showing curly dyschromic alterations. (Courtesy of Dr. González Otero.)

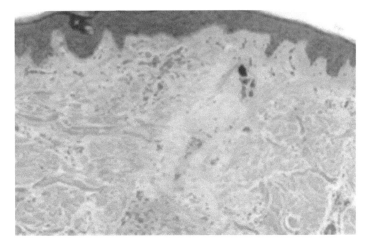

FIGURE 2.36 Histological aspect of ichthyosis of patient with Conradi-Hünermann syndrome. (Courtesy of Dr. González Otero.)

Pure Hair and Nail Ectodermal Dysplasia

Usually familial generalized hypotrichoses involve the body and scalp (Marie Unna, Jeanselme and Rime, Patjas, Bentley-Phillips and Grace types). Only the Spanish family described by Toribio and Quiñones (hereditary hypotrichosis simplex of the scalp) demonstrated normal body hair and involvement limited to the scalp. The two families we studied seem to be reverse images of hereditary hypotrichosis simplex of the scalp. They exhibited sparse body hair in contrast to abundant scalp hair mimicking uncombable hair.

Pure ectodermal dysplasias are developmental disorders affecting only tissues of ectodermal origin. Two pure ectodermal dysplasias involving only hair and nails have been described to date. Barbareschi et al. [46] describe congenital nail dystrophy and hypotrichosis associated with folliculitis decalvans in a family and suggest AD transmission. The authors reported peculiar clinical and ultrastructural hair findings that fit poorly into previously described conditions. They suggest that their patients may represent a new type of pure ectodermal dysplasia.

In 1998 [47], we had the opportunity to study two families with the following clinical findings:

1. Diffuse corporal hypotrichosis with multiple small hamartomatous anagenic follicles manifested at puberty
2. Significant involvement of eyebrows and eyelashes
3. Uncombable hair since childhood with no pili canaliculi
4. AD inheritance
5. Lack of other ectodermal cutaneous, nail, or mental involvement
6. Absence of significant findings from laboratory or endocrinological investigation

We therefore proposed familial pure hair dysplasia as a term for distinguishing the new condition from the pure hair and nail dysplasia described by the Italian group. Our patients appear to be reverse images of the hereditary hypotrichosis simplex of the scalp noted above: sparse body hair, abundant scalp hair mimicking uncombable hair with no pili canaliculi visible under scanning electron microscopy (Figures 2.37 through 2.40).

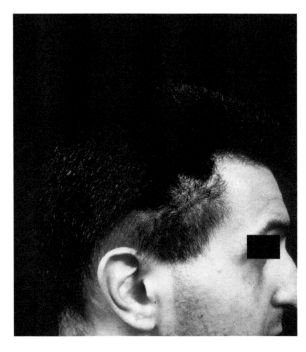

FIGURE 2.37   Pure hair and nail ectodermal dysplasia and diffuse hypotrichosis of scalp. (Courtesy of Dr. S. Cambiaghi.)

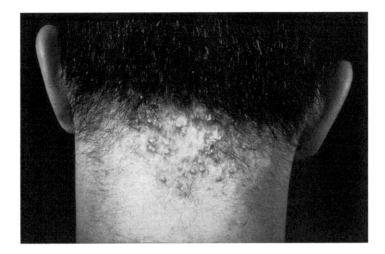

FIGURE 2.38   Occipital folliculitis decalvans.

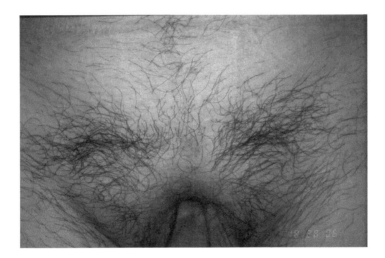

FIGURE 2.39   Pubic diffuse hypotrichosis.

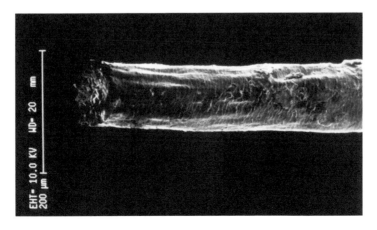

FIGURE 2.40   Branch-of-dry-wood appearance under scanning electron microscope.

Generalized Hamartoma of Hair Shaft Follicles

This hamartoma is a diffuse congenital malformation of the pilosebaceous follicles. Biopsies performed on any area reveal diverse and varied hamartomatous aspects. The disorder leads to atrichia or diffuse hypotrichosis that develops into alopecia totalis during adolescence. Approximately 20 cases have been described in the literature; most were sporadic processes in adults. Nevertheless, we had the opportunity to study three children from one family who were affected by this phenomenon as well as hyperelastic cutis and cystic fibrosis of the pancreas. The complications associated with the latter led to their deaths [48].

Generalized hamartoma of the hair shaft follicle is usually associated with immunological disorders such as myasthenia gravis, antinuclear antibodies, acetylcholine anti-receptor antibodies, and occasionally aminoaciduria. Localized forms have been described. Clinical observation reveals atrichia or diffuse hypotrichosis along with small papules or minimum cysts of follicular size on the face and signs of follicular atrophoderma on the trunk.

> **Histology:** Images of complex hamartomas of the pilosebaceous follicles similar to trichoepithelioma can be observed on any part of the body subjected to biopsy, especially of hairy areas and follicular lesions (Figures 2.41 and 2.42).
>
> **Clinical diagnosis:** Atrichia or progressive hypotrichosis with follicular atrophoderma and small papules or follicular cysts similar to milia are present. The disorder is usually associated with myasthenia gravis.
>
> **Laboratory analysis:** Antinuclear antibodies and acetylcholine anti-receptor may be found. Patients may present with aminoaciduria.

Non-Hereditary Congenital Hypotrichosis Simplex

We have observed children whose parents report diffuse congenital hypotrichosis since birth not associated with any sign of ectodermal or mesodermal dysplasia. Surprisingly, in some patients with "poor hair," this condition tends to improve with topical minoxidil (1 to 2%).

> **Clinical picture:** Usual patients are girls between 3 and 9 years of age who exhibit sparse growth of thin, fine hair and diffuse alopecia simulating female pattern androgenetic alopecia since birth (Figure 2.43). All medical and laboratory tests and trichograms appear normal.
>
> **Differential diagnosis:** Familial atrichia and congenital hypotrichoses (Kenue and Al-Dhafri, Jeanselme and Rime, and Marie Unna conditions) and various types of ectodermal and mesodermal disease groups should be ruled out [49]. Loose anagen and short anagen hair conditions also need to be ruled out.
>
> **Treatment:** In most cases, 1 to 2% minoxidil may improve this condition in a few months. Patients may recover partial or even total thickness and density of hair in a few years.

In summary, non-hereditary congenital hypotrichosis simplex [50] is a benign ectodermal or mesodermal dysplasia that is not familial or associated with any hair dysplasia. It appears predominantly in young girls and tends to improve with topical minoxidil. The etiology may be related to a delay of maturation of the pilosebaceous follicles of the scalp.

Conclusions

The psychological and cosmetic importance of hair is immense in our society. Disruption in the normal appearance of hair can predispose an individual to low self-esteem and negative body image. A detailed clinical history and examination accompanied by hair microscopy are essential for accurate diagnosis of a hair condition. In pediatric hair disorders, it is important that the parents are given a clear

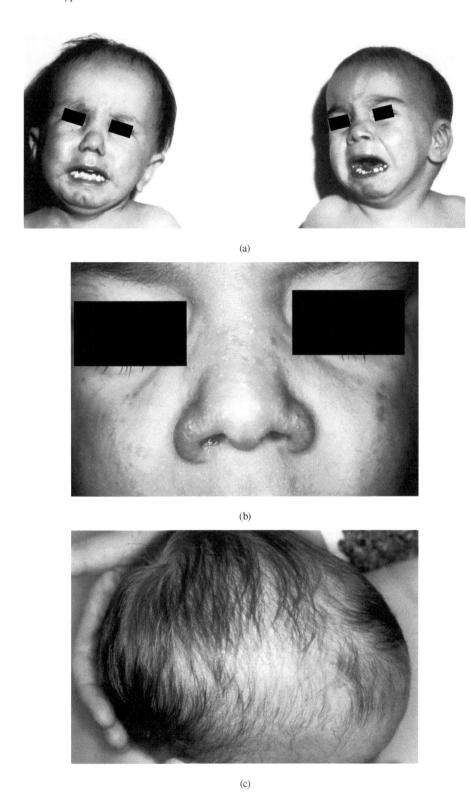

(a)

(b)

(c)

FIGURE 2.41 (a) Congenital generalized follicular hamartoma in two siblings. (b) Detail of papules on the face. (c) Generalized and unspecific hypotrichosis.

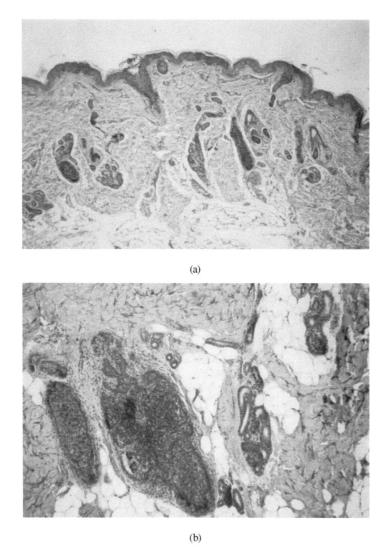

(a)

(b)

FIGURE 2.42   (a) Generalized hamartomatous hair follicles. (b) Detail of hamartoma.

understanding of the etiology and natural history of the disease and are offered genetic counseling if the disease is hereditary.

Unfortunately, no effective reliable therapies are available for many hair disorders. Treatment of hair conditions is mandatory in reversible conditions such as infections. Some conditions are amenable to surgical correction. Cosmetic solutions such as wigs can provide satisfactory camouflage if surgery is not an option and medical therapies fail.

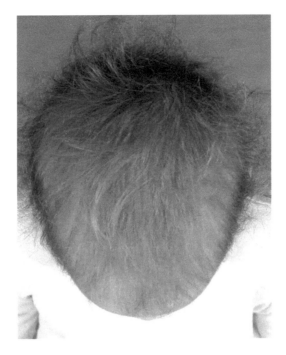

FIGURE 2.43 Three-year-old girl with non-familial (neither hair nor ectodermal) dysplasia-associated diffuse hypotrichosis.

REFERENCES

1. Bonnet R. Ueber hypotrichosis congenital universalis. *Anatomishe Hefte* 1892: 1–233.
2. Cockayne AE. *Inherited Abnormalities of the Skin and Its Appendages.* Oxford: Oxford University Press, 1933, p. 229.
3. Muller SA. Alopecia: syndromes of genetic significance. *J Invest Dermatol* 60: 475–492, 1975.
4. Sâlamon T. Hypotrichosis and alopecia in cases of genodermatosis. In *Hair Research Status and Future Aspects.* Berlin: Springer, 1981, pp. 396–407.
5. Betz RC, Cabral RM, Christiano AM, and Sprecher E. Unveiling the roots of monogenic genodermatosis: genotrichoses as a paradigm. *J Invest Dermatol* 132: 906–914, 2012.
6. Camacho F. Genodermatosis with hyptrichosis. In *Tricology.* Madrid: Aula Médica, 1996, pp. 219–236.
7. Boni R, Boni RH, Tsambaos D, Spycher MA, and Trueb RM. Trichorhinophalangeal syndrome. *Dermatology* 190: 152–155, 1995.
8. Lu FL, Hou JW, Tsai WS, Teng RJ et al. Trichorhinophalangeal syndrome type II associated with epiglottic aplasia and congenital nephrotic syndrome. *J Formos Med Assn* 96: 217–221, 1997.
9. Itin PH, Bohn S, Mathys D, Guggenheim R et al. Trichorhinophalangeal syndrome type III. *Dermatology* 193: 349–352, 1996.
10. Paradisi M, Angelo C, Conti G, Mostaccioli S et al. Dubowitz syndrome with keloidal lesions. *Clin Exp Dermatol* 19: 425–427, 1994.
11. Vadiakas G, Oulis C, Tsianos E, and Mavridou S. A typical Hallermann-Streiff syndrome in a 3-year-old child. *J Clin Pediatr Dent* 20: 63–68, 1995.
12. Fonseca MA and Mueller WA. Hallermann-Streiff syndrome: case report and recommendations for dental care. *ASDC J Dent Child* 61: 334–337, 1994.
13. Mandt N, Vogt A, and Blume-Peytabi U. Differential diagnosis of hair loss in children. *JDDG* 2: 399–411, 2004.
14. Freire-Maia N. Ectodermal dysplasia revisited. *Acta Genet Med Gemellol* (Roma) 26: 121–131, 1977.
15. Solomon LM and Keuer EJ. The ectodermal dysplasias. *Arch Dermatol* 116: 1295–1299, 1980.

16. Jones EM, Hersh JH, and Yusk JW. Aplasia cutis congenita, cleft palate, epidermolysis bullosa and ectrodactyly: a new syndrome? *Pediatr Dermatol* 9: 293–297, 1992.

17. Becker M, Rohrschneider K, Tilgen W, Weber BH et al. Familial juvenile macular dystrophy with congenital hypotrichosis capitis. *Ophthalmology* 95: 233–240, 1998.

18. Shimomura Y. Congenital hair loss disorders: rare, but not too rare. *J Dermatol* 39: 3–10, 2012.

19. Blume-Peytavi U, Fohles J, Schulz R, Wortmann G et al. Hypotrichosis, hair structure defects, hypercysteine hair and glucosuria: a new genetic syndrome? *Br J Dermatol* 134: 319–324, 1996.

20. Cáceres-Ríos H, Tamayo-Sanchez L, Duran-McKinster C, de la Luz Orozco M et al. Keratitis, ichthyosis, and deafness (KID syndrome): review of the literature and proposal of a new terminology. *Pediatr Dermatol* 13: 105–113, 1996.

21. Michaëlsson G, Olsson E, and Westermark P. The Rombo syndrome: a familial disorder with vermiculate atrophoderma, milia, hypotrichosis, trichoepitheliomas, basal cell carcinomas and peripheral vasodilation with cyanosis. *Acta Derm Venereol* 61: 497–503, 1981.

22. Ashinoff R, Jacobson M, and Belsito DV. Rombo syndrome: a second case report and review. *J Am Acad Dermatol* 28: 1011–1014, 1993.

23. Lacombe D and Taieb A. Overlap between the Bazex syndrome and congenital hypotrichosis and milia. *Am J Med Genet* 56: 423–424, 1995.

24. Kidd A, Carson L, Gregory DW, de Silva D et al. A Scottish family with Bazex-Dupre-Christol syndrome: follicular atrophoderma, congenital hypotrichosis, and basal cell carcinoma. *J Med Genet* 33: 493–497, 1996.

25. Goeteyn M, Geerts ML, Kint A, and De Weert J. The Bazex-Dupre-Christol syndrome. *Arch Dermatol* 130: 337–342, 1994.

26. Ferrando J and Grimalt R. Hereditary simple hypotrichosis. In *Atlas of Paediatric Trichology*. Madrid: Aula Médica, 2000, pp. 64–65.

27. Toribio J and Quiñones PA. Hereditary hypotrichosis simplex of the scalp: evidence for autosomal dominant inheritance. *Br J Dermatol* 91: 687–696, 1974.

28. Lestringant GG, Kuster W, Frossard PM, and Happle R. Congenital ichthyosis, follicular atrophoderma, hypotrichosis, and hypohidrosis: a new genodermatosis? *Am J Med Genet* 75: 186–189, 1998.

29. Steijlen PM, Neumann HA, der Kinderen DJ, Smeets DF et al. Congenital atrichia, palmoplantar hyperkeratosis, mental retardation, and early loss of teeth in four siblings: a new syndrome? *J Am Acad Dermatol* 30: 893–898, 1994.

30. Basaran E, Yilmaz E, Alpsoy E, and Yilmaz GG. Keratoderma, hypotrichosis and leukonychia totalis: a new syndrome? *Br J Dermatol* 133: 636–638, 1995.

31. Devriendt K, Van den Berghe H, and Fryns JP. Alopecia–mental retardation syndrome associated with convulsions and hypergonadotropic hypogonadism. *Clin Genet* 49: 6–9, 1996.

32. Nothen MM, Cichon S, Vogt IR, Hemmer S et al. A gene for universal congenital alopecia maps to chromosome 8p21–22. *Am J Hum Genet* 62: 386–390, 1998.

33. Cichon S, Anker M, Vogt IR, Rohleder H et al. Cloning, genomic organisation, alternative transcripts and mutational analysis of the gene responsible for autosomal recessive universal congenital alopecia. *Hum Mol Genet* 7: 1671–1679, 1998.

34. Rapelanoro R, Taieb A, and Lacombe D. Congenital hypotrichosis and milia: report of a large family suggesting X–linked dominant inheritance. *Am J Med Genet* 52: 487–490, 1994.

35. Podjasek JO and Hand JL. Marie Unna hereditary hypotrichosis: case report and review of the literature. *Pediatr Dermatol* 28: 202–204, 2011.

36. Gobello T, Mazzanti C, Fileccia P, Didona B et al. X-linked dominant chondrodysplasia punctata (Happle syndrome) with uncommon symmetrical shortening of the tubular bones. *Dermatology* 191: 323–327, 1995.

37. Armstrong DK and Burrows D. Congenital triangular alopecia. *Pediatr Dermatol* 13: 394–396, 1996.

38. Yamakazi M, Irisawa R, and Tsuboi R. Temporal triangular alopecia and a review of 52 past cases. *J Dermatol* 37: 360–362, 2010.

39. García-Hernández MJ, Rodríguez-Pichardo A, and Camacho F. Congenital triangular alopecia (Brauer nevus). *Pediatr Dermatol* 12: 301–303, 1995.

40. Assouly P and Happle R. A hairy paradox: congenital triangular alopecia with a central hair tuft. *Dermatology* 221: 107–109, 2010.

41. Zapata HH, Sletten LJ, and Pierpont ME. Congenital cardiac malformations in Adams-Oliver syndrome. *Clin Genet* 47: 80–84, 1995.

42. Gershoni-Baruch R and Leibo R. Aplasia cutis congenita, high myopia, and cone–rod dysfunction in two sibs: a new autosomal recessive disorder. *Am J Med Genet* 61: 42–44, 1996.

43. Herve A, Maroteaux P, Denoix C, Wechsler J et al. Happle-type Conradi-Hünermann syndrome: a sporadic case. *Ann Dermatol Venereol* 118: 790–791, 1991.

44. Herd RM and Benton EC. Keratosis follicularis spinulosa decalvans: report of a new pedigree. *Br J Dermatol* 134: 138–142, 1996.

45. Harth W and Linse R. Keratosis follicularis spinulosa decalvans associated with patent ductus arteriosus and hypospadia in an Asiatic patient. *Hautarzt* 50: 295–298, 1999.

46. Barbareschi M, Cambiaghi S, Crupi AC, and Tadini G. Family with "pure" hair–nail ectodermal dysplasia. *Am J Med Genet* 72: 91–93, 1997.

47. Ferrando J, Grimalt R, Garcia Lora E et al. Familiar diffuse corporal hypotrichosis with uncombable hair: a familial "pure" hair dysplasia. 2nd Intercontinental Meeting of Hair Research Societies. Washington, DC, 1998.

48. Mascaro JM Jr, Ferrando J, Bombi JA et al. Congenital generalized follicular hamartoma associated with alopecia and cystic fibrosis in three siblings. *Arch Dermatol* 131: 454–458, 1995.

49. Solomon LM and Keuer EI. The ectodermal dysplasias: problems of classification and some newer syndromes. *Arch Dermatol* 116: 1295–1289, 1980.

50. Ferrando J and Grimalt R. Non-hereditary congenital hypotrichosis simplex (unpublished data).

3

Acquired Hair Disorders

This chapter considers a series of changes of hair due to color (e.g., green hair) or loss (alopecia) including cicatricial (tufted folliculitis) and non-cicatricial (alopecia areata, trichotillomania) forms that occur primarily during childhood and adolescence. We do not consider more common processes that are diagnosed easily, for example, androgenic alopecia or telogen and anagen effluvium. For further information on these processes, readers can consult the textbook by Camacho and co-workers [1] or the review of Moreno-Romero and Grimalt [2]. Deficient hair losses caused by nutritional or metabolic disorders are not addressed either. Finally, the descriptions include infrequent clinical patterns such as alopecia parvimaculata and bird's nest hair.

Transient Neonatal Hair Loss

Hair development begins in utero at the ninth week with the formation of follicular units composed of epidermally derived follicles and mesodermally derived papillae [3]. Primary hair follicles first develop on the eyebrows, upper lip, and chin. They later develop over the scalp in a frontal-to-occipital direction and over the body in a cephalocaudal direction. Secondary follicles then form at the sides of the primary follicles, producing typical groups of three hairs on a follicular unit. At 16 weeks' gestation, hair production begins in the follicles. All follicles produce lanugo hair that grows 2 to 3 cm in length [4]. Fine lanugo hair covers the scalp and appears elsewhere in a cephalocaudal direction, eventually covering the entire fetus. This constitutes the first anagen (growth) wave. At 26 to 28 weeks' gestation, the body and most of the scalp hair follicles enter catagen and subsequent telogen phases in a programmed wave in a cephalocaudal direction in the body and a frontal-to-parietal direction on the scalp. Most of these telogen hairs are shed in utero [5], although this may be delayed until after birth. A band-like area of occipital hair does not enter telogen until 8 to 12 weeks after birth. These occipital hairs fall out, producing a well-defined area of alopecia known as occipital alopecia of the newborn at 4 to 8 months of age [6]. This process has been renamed transient neonatal hair loss (TNHL) [7].

The duration of growth of the scalp hairs extends, while the duration of body hair growth shortens to produce hairs 1 cm in length. These second body hairs grow for 4 to 8 weeks, then enter telogen, and are shed during the first 3 or 4 months of life and are replaced by a third coat of hair. Body hairs progressively shorten into vellus hairs, most of which do not protrude from follicles. Scalp hair enlarges progressively with each cycle into terminal hair. Some infants display intermediate hair from 3 months until the age of 2 years. This hair is coarser than lanugo hairs, but still sparsely pigmented [8].

At full term of a pregnancy, the scalp reveals two consecutive waves of hair, each running from forehead to occiput. Toward the end of the first year of life, after development of the first two synchronized waves of telogen, the scalp undergoes a transition to a random mosaic pattern in which each hair has its own intrinsic rhythm. This asynchrony continues throughout life unless modified by pregnancy or illness.

Clinical diagnosis: A band-like area of occipital hypotrichosis appears until 8 to 12 weeks after birth: the occipital alopecia of the newborn is seen around 4 to 8 months of age (Figure 3.1).

Treatment: Spontaneous regrowing of hair is usual.

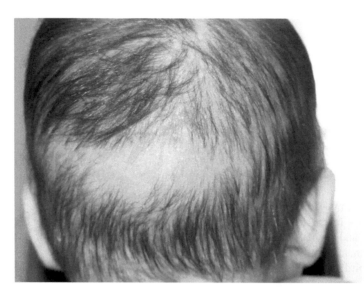

FIGURE 3.1   Transient neonatal hair loss with characteristic band-like hypotrichosis of the occipital area.

Focal and Multifocal Alopecia Areata

Alopecia areata (AA) is a chronic follicular inflammatory process of autoimmune origin that leads to interruption of the follicular cycle during an early phase of anagen with detachment of telogen hairs. Therefore, when the cause is no longer active, recovery is complete after an extended time (months or even years) has passed. AA appears in the form of one or several rounded, well-defined plaques of non-cicatricial alopecia that may evolve into alopecia totalis or alopecia universalis. Focal AA consists of localized forms of AA consisting of one or several plaques (multifocal AA) of ophiasic distribution around temporal and occipital areas.

Short hairs on the borders of the plaques measuring a few millimeters in length, thicker at the distal ends ("exclamation mark or peladic hairs"), are pathognomonic as are the "cadaveric" hairs seen as black points. These types of hairs indicate that the process is active and the plaques will extend even further. When recovery begins, fine white vellus hair is observed in the centers of the plaques.

AA is a frequent finding (approximately 2% of dermatological consultations) of familial incidence (in at least 25% of cases). It commonly begins in childhood and 60% of patients are under 20 years old. AA is chronic and relapsing, and involves several etiopathogenic factors such as foci of infections, stress, and presence of immune complexes or autoantibodies over a genetic base. Association with immunological disorders is frequent, especially with autoimmune thyroiditis, celiac disease, atopy, Down syndrome, vitiligo, and others [9]. In some of these disorders, evolution is chronic and the prognosis is poor.

We must also bear in mind that AA can affect the nails, and in cases of trachyonychia, the appearance of the nail plate is rough. An exceptional clinical pattern in children is the diffuse form of AA. It must be considered when diffuse acute alopecia is observed [10].

Clinical diagnosis: One or several rounded, well-defined plaques of non-cicatricial alopecia may show "exclamation mark hairs" (Figure 3.2) on their borders. These plaques develop chronically and tend to converge in ophiasic patterns in temporal areas. In the acute diffuse type of AA, peladic hairs are useful signs for supporting such a diagnosis. A differential diagnosis should consider congenital alopecia triangularis, alopecia parvimaculata, and trichotillomania.

Light microscopy: The peladic hairs or hairs that are easily detached from the plaque borders are of the telogen type (Figure 3.2).

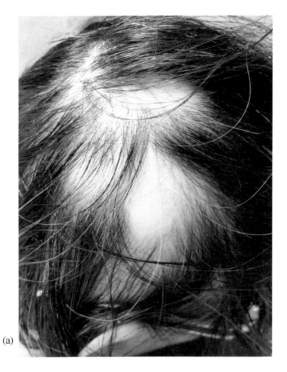

(a)

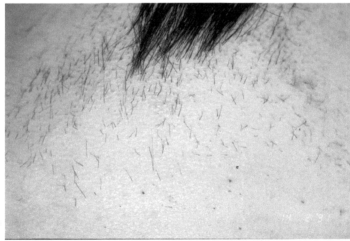

(b)

FIGURE 3.2 Multifocal alopecia areata. (a) Typical plaques of alopecia areata showing non-cicatricial rounded aspects. (b) Multiple peladic hairs on margins of plaques. (c) Detail of initial formation of peladic ("exclamation mark") hair: telogenic root and distal end with wider diameter. *(Continued)*

Dermoscopy: Peladic and "cadaveric" hairs (black dots) and lighter color dots that correspond to prominent sebaceous glands in empty follicles on the skin surface can be seen (Figure 3.3).

Histology: Biopsy of active borders of plaques shows moderate round cell peribulbar inflammatory infiltrate (Figure 3.4). A study with monoclonal antibodies shows that this infiltrate consists mostly of T-helper lymphocytes.

Treatment: The etiopathogenesis of AA has not been clarified completely. Several treatments may be helpful although individual responses to their use are quite variable. To ensure that side effects are reduced to a minimum, we suggest establishment of a scale that classifies treatments based on their levels of aggressiveness, while considering the patient's degree of complaint.

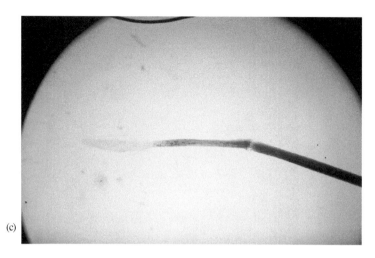

(c)

FIGURE 3.2 (Continued)   Multifocal alopecia areata. (a) Typical plaques of alopecia areata showing non-cicatricial rounded aspects. (b) Multiple peladic hairs on margins of plaques. (c) Detail of initial formation of peladic ("exclamation mark") hair: telogenic root and distal end with wider diameter.

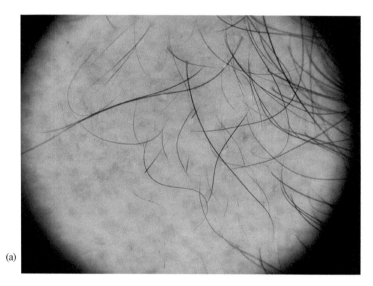

(a)

FIGURE 3.3   Trichoscopy results: (a) characteristic "exclamation mark hairs"; (b) black dots (cadaveric hairs); and (c) lighter dots representing empty hair follicles. *(Continued)*

In localized focal forms of AA (plaques, for example), we recommend local rubefacients only. In this phase, the plaques often undergo spontaneous involution. In multifocal AA, more aggressive treatments are usually necessary: 1 to 2% dithranol locally for short contact therapy or 2 to 3% minoxidil plus clobetasol propionate 0.025 to 0.050% topical solution (Figure 3.5) [11]. The oral administration of 10 mg per day of biotin may be helpful. In severe cases, steroid pulse therapy can be used [12]. Local sensitization with diphencyprone or dinitrochloroben-zene (DNCB) and steroid treatment is not recommended in children.

Alopecia Areata Totalis and Universalis

Alopecia areata totalis is an AA that affects the scalp. AA universalis affects all hair follicles of the body including eyebrows and eyelashes. Both forms are related to the extreme evolution of AA, although

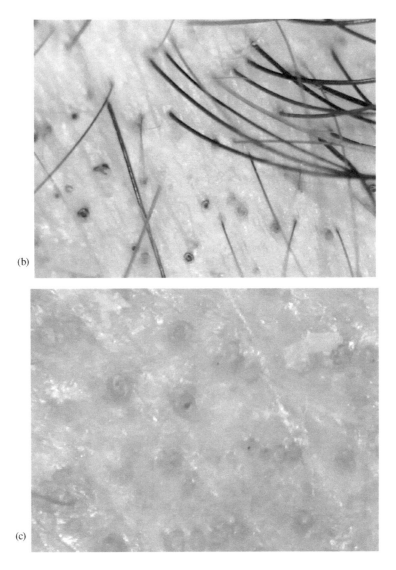

(b)

(c)

FIGURE 3.3 (Continued) Trichoscopy results: (a) characteristic "exclamation mark hairs"; (b) black dots (cadaveric hairs); and (c) lighter dots representing empty hair follicles.

they may begin with acute, diffuse forms. These generalized forms of AA are often associated with processes that have immunological bases, especially Hashimoto's thyroiditis, and others such as pernicious anemia, vitiligo, myasthenia gravis, and celiac disease in children [13]. Many patients are atopic, and in half of the cases the possibility of regrowth is not especially favorable. AA should be studied following a standardized assessment protocol such as that proposed by Olsen et al. [14].

Clinical diagnosis: Children, youths, and adults may be affected by chronic acquired alopecia totalis or alopecia universalis (Figure 3.6) developed from AA in plaques or rarely from acute diffuse AA. These alopecias may affect several members of the same family or community. Some advanced cases of alopecia totalis involve the entire area of the scalp with the exception of isolated hairs on the borders of the scalp and vertex. This condition may be accompanied by trachyonychia (Figure 3.7) or associated with immunological diseases. A differential diagnosis must consider atrichias and hypotrichoses (congenital alopecias) [14].

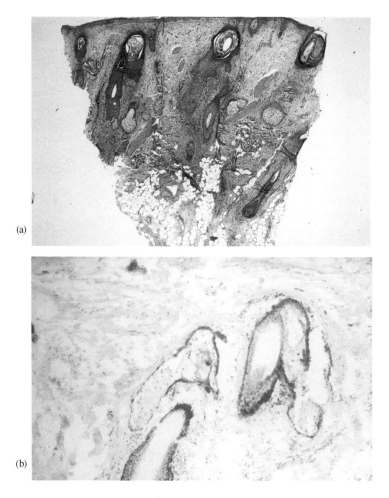

(a)

(b)

FIGURE 3.4   Histopathology: (a) perifollicular peribulbar infiltrate (POF); (b) characteristic CD4 positive.

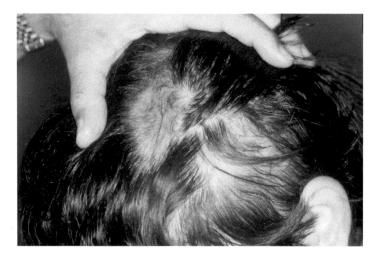

FIGURE 3.5   New hair appears after short contact dithranol therapy.

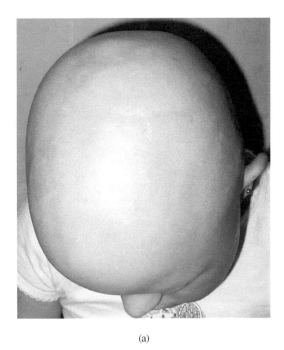

(a)

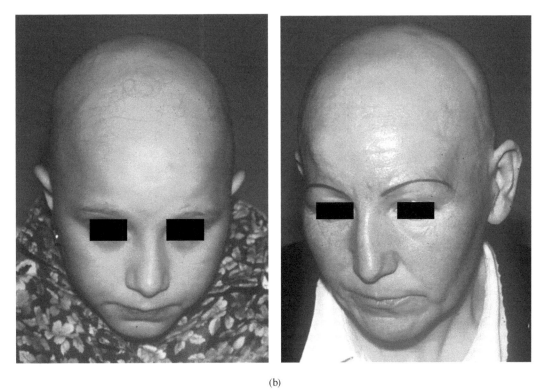

(b)

FIGURE 3.6 Alopecia areata totalis and universalis. (a) Alopecia areata totalis partially spares the eyebrows, eyelashes, and other body hair. Alopecia areata universalis affects eyebrows and eyelashes. (b) Familial alopecia areata universalis.

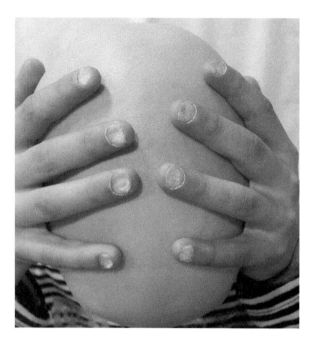

FIGURE 3.7   Trachyonychia: sanded aspect of nails associated with alopecia areata.

Laboratory analysis: A slightly increased rate of circulating immune complexes and positive reaction to some types of antitissue antibodies with low counts are common. In thyroiditis, the number of antithyroid antibodies is especially high, and alterations of T4 and TSH occur. The IgE level may be high in atopic individuals.

Dermoscopy: Peladic and cadaveric hairs and yellow dots are present.

Histology: Minimal peribulbar lymphocytic infiltrates are observed.

Treatment: The first step is control of an underlying disease. Second, irritant topical treatments should be employed such as short contact therapy with dithranol (1 to 2%) or a diphencyprone course [15]; in both cases approximately 30% of patients respond. A 2 to 3% solution of min-oxidil with clobetasol propionate 0.025 to 0.05% in topical solution is currently recommended as well as a pulsed corticotherapy with methylprednisolone in severe cases [12,15–17].

Trichotillomania

Trichotillomania is the compulsive habit of consciously or unconsciously pulling out hair that causes limited or widespread areas of irregular alopecia that do not follow a characteristic pattern. This disorder may also affect the eyebrows and eyelashes. During childhood, trichotillomania is related to nervous tics. In adolescents and adults, it may represent a true neurosis. It is an expression of a personal conflict within a family (overprotective mother, passive father, competition between siblings, lack of attention) or in a social (emotional relationship) environment.

Trichotillomania is found in children, adolescents, and adult women who have the habit of rolling their hair between their fingers. It is more frequent in females and the older the age, the greater the severity. The areas least affected are those that are difficult to reach, for example the vertex and nape of the neck. This is why the condition affects upper eyelashes and not the lower ones. It is often associated with trichophagia and bulimia [18,19]. Four variants of trichotillomania have been described.

Trichotemnomania (from the Greek *temnein* meaning *to cut*) is hair loss due to cutting or shaving in the context of obsessive–compulsive disorder. Trichotemnomania is not purely voluntary; it is performed to relieve stress. Although the cutting or shaving is a conscious act, patients are resistant to admitting to their habit. They may be embarrassed by their appearance and have feelings of guilt. The hair is usually cut with a scissors or shaved. The diagnostic key is the presence of follicle openings with filled hair shafts on a healthy-looking scalp [20].

Another type of artificial hair loss resulting from perpetual rubbing of the scalp that causes fracturing of hair shafts is **trichoteiromania**. The patient presents with bald spots within hair of different lengths; the hair may appear similar to hair cut with scissors. White tips are seen at the ends of the shafts in the form of distal splitting.

A type of hair loss with associated psychiatric comorbidity is **trichodaganomania**, characterized by the compulsive habit of biting one's own hair. In adults, a very selective type of trichophagia called **trichorrhizophagia** was reported. The patient ate the roots of the hairs he plucked [21].

Clinical diagnosis: Patients are children, adolescents, and females with tense familial relationships who show irregular plaques of non-cicatricial alopecia that do not follow a characteristic pattern. Hair of variable lengths and thickness is observed within the same area on the scalp (Figure 3.8) and on the eyebrows and upper eyelashes (Figure 3.9). Peladic or cadaveric hairs are never found. Trichotemnomania must be differentiated primarily from the diffuse forms of AA in plaques.

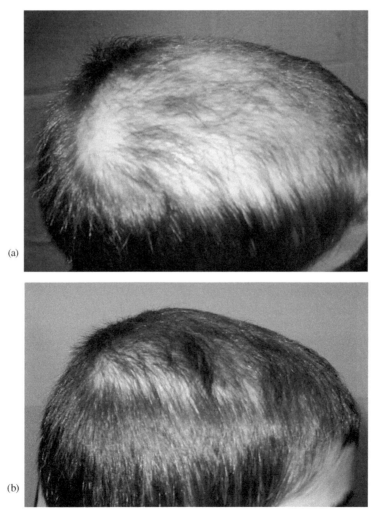

(a)

(b)

FIGURE 3.8 Trichotillomania. (a) Typical aspect of hair with irregular plaques of variable length and thickness. On close examination, hairs appear cut; the plaques do not follow a characteristic pattern. (b) Same patient after treatment with oral N-acetyl-cysteine.

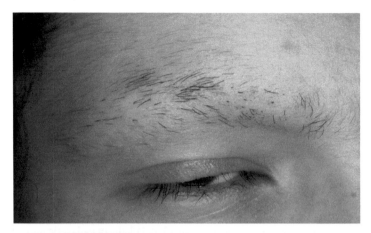

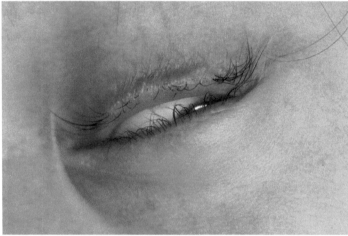

FIGURE 3.9   Similar aspect of the eyebrows. The alopecic area is not homogeneous and regular in the eyelashes as it is with alopecia areata; upper eyelashes are obviously more affected.

Light microscopy: Most of the roots are anagen types since the telogen hairs are obviously the first to become detached.

Histology: In doubtful cases, histology is very useful. In the initial phases, hemorrhages and intrafollicular and perifollicular fissures are present. The advanced phases are characterized by perifollicular fibrosis and occasionally granulomas. Empty hair canals and trichomalacia (injured follicles with finely twisted hairs) are characteristic signs.

Treatment: An attempt should be made to determine whether the problem is of psychological origin and resolve it. In children, resolution may involve reducing the pressures and demands made by parents, increasing confidence and promoting positive attitudes, prescribing shampoos and placebo, and careful examination during each visit. The participation of a psychiatrist is usually required for adults and adolescents. A new treatment with oral N-acetyl-cysteine has been launched successfully [22].

Alopecia Parvimaculata

This alopecia exhibits small cicatricial plaques (atrophic with angular borders) and is acute and epidemic in communities of children such as summer camps and schools. Its exact cause is not known; mycotic and bacterial infections have been ruled out [23]. Histologically, it usually shows cicatricial changes with atrophy and fibrosis. Nevertheless, many cases recover within a few months. In other cases, the histology is compatible with that of AA.

The limited number of studies on this subject discusses cases within the same children's community, although we observed several sporadic cases involving chronic relapsing evolution. Whether this alopecia is a true nosologic entity; represents a clinical form of AA in children when clinical data, histology, and evolution are compatible; corresponds to a pseudopelade (compatible histology and chronic non-recoverable evolution); or is a fungal or bacterial post-infection cicatricial alopecia not noticed earlier and no longer reported [13] is questionable.

Clinical diagnosis: This condition always involves children who present with several small plaques (0.5 to 1.5 cm) on the scalp. The plaques may be acute (several cases found in the same child community) or insidious, chronic, and relapsing (sporadic) cases. The plaques usually have slightly depressed centers without peladic hair and borders with irregular angles (Figure 3.10). Usually the patient has no history of prior infection, traumas, or bites.

Histology: Alopecia parvimaculata generally is compatible with a cicatricial-type alopecia, although sometimes it is referred to as AA.

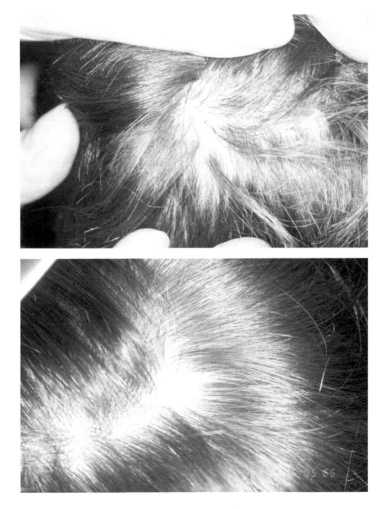

FIGURE 3.10   Alopecia parvimaculata exhibits small, irregular alopecic patches with central atrophic aspects and angular borders.

Tufted Folliculitis

This chronic dermatosis of the scalp is characterized by one or several plaques of cicatricial alopecia in which several locks of hair emerge from a single common hair channel [24,25]. This is a chronic process that begins with a local inflammatory pattern with erythema, edema, exudation, pustules, scabs, and desquamation. It is accompanied by pruritus and/or pain, occasionally with inflammatory regional adenopathy. Evolution occurs in outbreaks. Although bacterial microorganisms, primarily *Staphylococcus aureus*, are often found in microbiological cultures, the condition does not respond to systemic or topical antibiotic treatment.

Biopsies show several hairs in a single hair channel with intense perifollicular inflammatory infiltrates of round cells and neutrophils on the superior and mid dermis. Granulomas and follicular rupture are also observed. Following the intense follicular damage caused by the pulling effect, the hair is grouped in a single channel formed by the ruptures of several neighboring pilosebaceous follicles [26,27].

Tufted folliculitis is found primarily in adolescents and young adults, and evolves into cicatricial alopecia. Its etiology is unknown although perhaps local malformative nevoid factors lead to the superinfection of plaques post puberty. Traumatic factors may also be involved. The disorder may be associated with acne keloidalis of the nape.

> **Clinical diagnosis:** Adolescents and young adults show one or several chronic inflammatory plaques in which the hair emerges in the form of tufts (Figure 3.11). Dermoscopy allows us to observe the common emerging of hair from a channel more accurately (Figure 3.12). Mycology is negative and bacteriological examination shows growth of *S. aureus*. The choice locations are the parietal and occipital regions. Tufted folliculitis is more common in males.
>
> **Histology:** As shown in Figure 3.13, inflammatory infiltrates of rounded neutrophils and histiocyte and plasma cells in a perifollicular location on the superior and mid dermis. Giant cell granuloma and destruction of the follicular walls joining several follicles and forming a single hair channel occupied by several hairs are characteristic.
>
> **Treatment:** Tufted folliculitis does not respond to topical or systemic antibiotics. Some cases respond to oral fusidic acid or oral retinoids. Topical 3% solution of indomethacin is usually helpful. Surgical removal has been indicated for small plaques.

Bird's Nest Hair

Bird's nest hair is tangling of the hair primarily caused by piling long hair on top of the head and massaging it with shampoo. This phenomenon of tangles that create a thick, dense mass of intermingled hair has been observed in children and young girls who have not shown previous hair alterations. Lifting a child's hair on top of his or her head during bathing or shampooing will cause matting. The improper use of shampoos, especially cationic types, leads to increased roughness of the squamae of the hair cuticles that become intermingled and tangled with other hairs until they form a viscous, matted mass [28,29]. In most cases it is impossible to untangle the result even with capillary conditioners. The only possible solution is to cut the hair in the area affected. Bird's nest hair may occur in normal hair.

> **Clinical diagnosis:** Common patients are young and adolescent girls who show pronounced tangling of the hair in a specific area that looks like a bun. The hair is impossible to brush or comb and the tangled mass of hair cannot be undone (Figure 3.14).
>
> **Light microscopy:** The main finding is a viscous mass of intermingled hair (Figure 3.15).
>
> **Scanning electron microscopy:** The viscous mass phenomenon can be observed and the images show the adherence of hairs into a viscous amorphous mass.
>
> **Treatment:** Hair should be washed as it falls normally, not pulled to the top of the head. Patients should use plenty of conditioner every time they shampoo.

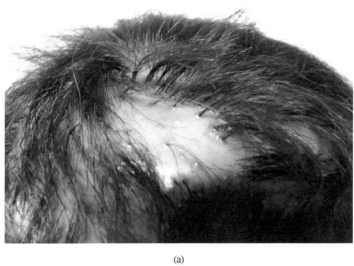

(a)

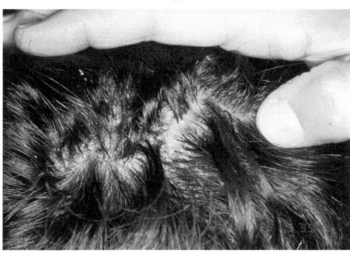

(b)

FIGURE 3.11 Tufted folliculitis. (a) Typical clinical aspects: grouped hairs emerging from inflammatory patches of scalp. (b) Same aspect in a fully developed case.

Green Hair

Green hair is a dyschromia characterized by green color. It is found in young people with fair or blonde hair as a sporadic and acquired form. Green hair is caused by insoluble copper deposits that fix to hair cortex with a priori damage to the cuticles [30, 31].

Green hair usually originates from direct contact with domestic water or swimming pool water with high copper content. The copper is released by different mechanisms. In domestic water, copper concentration increases when the pH decreases due to water fluoridation. The use of copper-based algicides in swimming pools also increases the copper in the water. In all cases, prior damage to cuticles seems essential. Hair damage may be of physical (heat, intense sun exposure, compulsive brushing) or chemical origin (bleaching agents, dyes, permanent waves, alkaline shampoos).

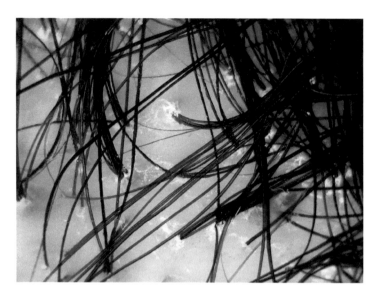

FIGURE 3.12   Dermoscopy observation. Hairs emerging from common follicular channel in old case without perifollicular inflammation.

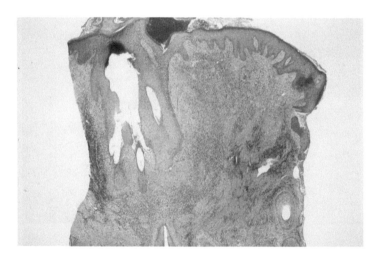

FIGURE 3.13   Dense perifollicular infiltrates. Detail of the infiltrate reveals foreign body granulomas joining several neighboring follicles in a single follicular channel.

Green hair may also be caused by using shampoo with a tar or copper base. Workers in the metal (copper, nickel, cobalt, chromium) industries are often affected. Other causes are use of preparations with yellow mercury oxide bases to treat tinea capitis; wearing headgear made with copper metal components; and extravasation of serum containing dipyridamole [31,32].

> **Clinical diagnosis:** Children and adolescents with fair or blonde hair exhibit one or several locks of green colored hair (Figure 3.16). They normally frequent swimming pools where similar cases can be found.
>
> **Scanning electron microscopy:** Hair is detached from the cuticle, leaving the cortex completely exposed (Figure 3.17).
>
> **X-ray microanalysis:** An increase in the copper fraction can be observed in both the green hair and also in hair with normal color [33]; see Figure 3.18.

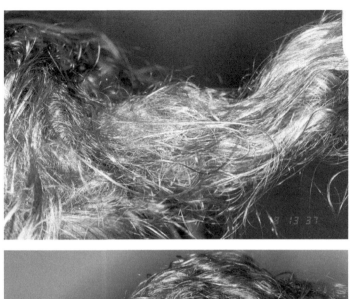

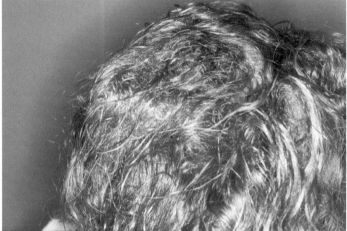

FIGURE 3.14 Bird's nest hair is tangled and impossible to brush or comb.

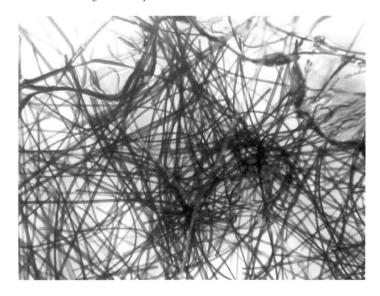

FIGURE 3.15 Intermingled mass of hairs viewed under microscope.

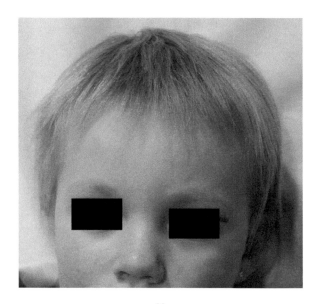

(a)

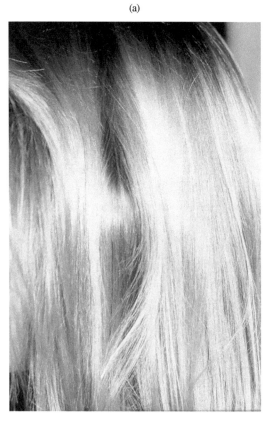

(b)

FIGURE 3.16   Green hair. (a) Of a child after swimming season. (b) Severe case in a young girl.

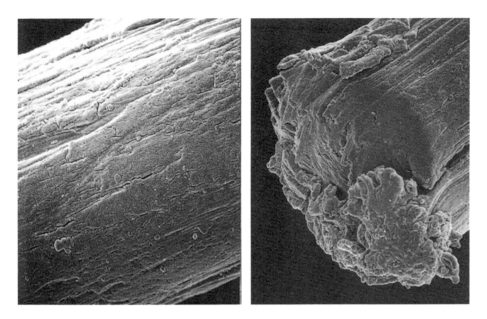

FIGURE 3.17 Scanning electron microscope image shows weathering of cuticles in both normal and green hair of the same patient. (Source: Mascaró J.M. Jr. et al. Green hair. *Cutis* 56: 37–40, 1995. With permission.)

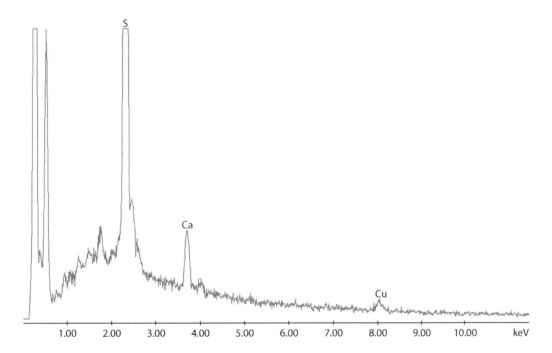

FIGURE 3.18 X-ray microanalysis showing marked copper peak.

Treatment: D-penicillamine-based shampoo (250 mg D-penicillamine + 5 ml water + 5 ml shampoo) is recommended. Application of 1.5% aqueous solution of 1-hydroxiethyl diphosphonic acid and immersion of hair in a 3% hydrogen peroxide solution are also effective. The first treatment to try should be a careful rinse in lemon juice; a second choice would be vinegar. The acidity of lemon juice or vinegar will remove most of the green color.

REFERENCES

1. Camacho FM, Tosti A, Randall VA, and Price VH. *Montagna Trichology*, Madrid: Aula Médica, 2016.
2. Moreno-Romero JA and Grimalt R. Hair loss in infancy. *G Ital Dermatol Venereol* 149: 55–78, 2014.
3. Harrison S and Sinclair R. Optimal management of hair loss [alopecia] in children. *Am J Clin Dermatol* 4: 757–770, 2003.
4. Lavker RM, Bertolino AP, Klein LM et al. Biology of hair follicles. In *Dermatology in General Medicine*, 5th ed. Boston: McGraw-Hill, 1993, pp. 230–238.
5. Cutrone M and Grimalt R. Where has all that hair gone? *Clin Exp Dermatol* 31: 136–137, 2006.
6. Olsen E. Hair disorders. In *Textbook of Pediatric Dermatology*, 2nd ed. Oxford: Blackwell, 2006, pp. 1753–1822.
7. Cutrone M and Grimalt R. Transient neonatal hair loss. *Eur J Pediatr* 164: 630–632, 2005.
8. Sinclair RD, Banfield CC, and Dawber RP. Hair structure and function. In *Handbook of Diseases of the Hair and Scalp*. Oxford: Blackwell, 1999, pp. 3–23.
9. Todes-Taylor N, Turner R, Wood G et al. T cell subpopulations in alopecia areata. *J Am Acad Dermatol* 11: 216–223, 1984.
10. Sinclair RP, Banfield CC, and Dawber RPR, Eds. *Handbook of Diseases of the Hair and Scalp*. Oxford: Blackwell, 1999.
11. Shapiro J and Price VH. Hair regrowth: therapeutic agents. *Dermatol Clin* 16: 341–356, 1998.
12. Sharma VK and Muralidhar S. Treatment of widespread alopecia areata in young patients with monthly oral corticosteroid pulse. *Pediatr Dermatol* 15: 313–317, 1998.
13. Rook A and Dawber R, Eds. *Diseases of the Hair and Scalp*. Oxford: Blackwell, 1991.
14. Olsen E, Hordinsly M, McDonald-Hull S et al. Alopecia areata investigational assessment guidelines. *J Am Acad Dermatol* 40: 242–246, 1999.
15. Tosti A, Guidetti MS, Bardazzi F et al. Long-term results of topical immunotherapy in children with alopecia totalis or alopecia universalis. *J Am Acad Dermatol* 35: 199–201, 1996.
16. Price V. Topical minoxidil in extensive alopecia areata, including a 3-year follow up. *Dermatologica* 175 Suppl. 2: 36–41, 1987.
17. Shapiro J and Price VH. Hair regrowth: therapeutic agents. *Dermatol Clin* 16: 341–356, 1998.
18. Müller SA. Obsessive-compulsive disorder: trichotillomania. *Dermatol Clin* 5: 595–601, 1987.
19. Weillard DS. The clinical evaluation of pathologic hair loss with a diagnostic sign in trichotillomania. *Cutis* 24: 293–301, 1979.
20. Orgaz-Molina J, Husein-El Ahmed H, Soriano-Hernández MI et al. Trichotemnomania: hair loss mediated by a compulsive habit not admitted by patients. *Acta Dermatol Venereol* 92: 183–184, 2012.
21. Grimalt R and Happle R. Trichorrhizophagia. *Eur J Dermatol* 14: 266–267, 2004.
22. Goulding JM. N-acetylcysteine in trichotillomania: further thoughts. *Br J Dermatol*. 2015. February 1. doi: 10.1111/bjd.13693.
23. Höfer W. Sporadisches Auftreten von Alopecia parvimacularis. *Dermatol Wochenschr* 149: 381, 1964.
24. Pujol RM, Matías-Guiu X, García-Patos V et al. Tufted-hair folliculitis. *Clin Exp Dermatol* 16: 199–201, 1991.
25. Luelmo-Aguilar J, González-Castro U, and Castells-Rodellas A. Tufted folliculitis: a study of four cases. *Br J Dermatol* 128: 454–457, 1993.
26. Veraldi S, Grimalt R, Cappio F et al. Tufted-hair follilculitis. *Eur J Dermatol* 5: 125–127, 1995.
27. Campo-Voegeli A, Ferrando J, Grimalt R et al. Foliculitis en penachos: una forma clinic-patológica de alopecia cicatricial. *Piel* 11: 511–515, 1994.
28. Dawber RWP and Calman CD. Bird's nest hair: matting of the scalp hair due to shampooing. *Clin Exp Dermatol* 1: 155–158, 1976.
29. Howell RG. Matting of the hair by shampoo. *Br J Dermatol* 68: 99, 1956.
30. Gould D, Slater DN, and Durrat TE. A case of green hair: a consequence of exogenous copper and permanent waving. *Clin Exp Dermatol* 9: 545–553, 1984.
31. Stidierling M and Christophers E. Why hair turns green. *Acta Dermatol Venereol* 73: 321–322, 1993.
32. Alegre V, Botella-Estrada R, Sanmartín O et al. El hombre del pelo verde. *Piel* 6: 513–514, 1991.
33. Mascaró JM Jr, Ferrando J, Fontarnau R et al. Green hair. *Cutis* 56: 37–40, 1995.

Glossary

Alopecia: Acquired hair loss.

Atrichia: Congenital absence of hair.

Bamboo hair: See trichorrhexis invaginata.

Bird's nest hair: Intense tangling or matting without knots as a result of improper handling.

Bubble hair: Acquired anomaly of the hair shaft due to the presence of air bubbles inside the shaft, usually caused by excessive dry heat or due to the direct application of heat to damp hair.

Cadaveric hairs: Short hairs resembling dots found at the margins of active plaques of alopecia areata.

Corkscrew hair: Atypical acquired form of pili torti clinically characterized by thick, dark scalp hairs that coil into a unique double spiral.

Exclamation mark hair: See peladic hair.

Golf tee hair: Peculiar deformation of the distal end of a hair shaft after breakage in trichorrhexis invaginata; a trichological marker of Netherton syndrome.

Green hair: Peculiar hair color due to the accumulation of extrinsic copper in the hair shaft.

Hypotrichosis: Congenital diffuse absence of hair.

Kinky hair: Complex hair dysplasia including atypical images of pili torti, trichorrhexis nodosa and/or monilethrix; considered a marker of Menkes syndrome.

Loose anagen hair: Peculiar condition characterized by the easy pluckability of anagen hair without pain; ruffling of the proximal cuticle is also present.

Monilethrix: Dominant hereditary defect characterized by regular periodic constrictions in the hair shaft that result in fiber breakage a few millimeters from the point where they emerge from the scalp.

Ophiasic pattern: Serpiginous pattern of alopecia at the peripheral margins of the scalp characteristic of some chronic forms of alopecia areata.

Peladic hair (exclamation mark hair): Short hair that is thinner near the root and found at the margins of active plaques of alopecia areata.

Pili annulati (ringed hair): Alternating dilations of the medulla; hair appears ringed or spangled.

Pili canaliculi: Longitudinal grooves usually seen in a clinical condition called uncombable hair. In a transverse section under scanning electron microscopy, the hair shaft shows a kidney appearance or triangular aspect (pili trianguli).

Pili torti: Hair fibers show regular and often abrupt twists; can be an inherited familial trait and may be a component of various different syndromes (Beare, Crandall, Bazex, Björnstad).

Pili trianguli: Triangular aspect of hair shaft section typically seen in uncombable hair.

Pseudomonilethrix: Artefact that appears as a series of flat nodes caused by incorrect handling of hair; familial cases have been described as idiopathic hair fragility.

Ringed hair: See pili annulati.

Ruffling: Regular spiral detachment of the inner root sheath, usually but not exclusively found in loose anagen hair syndrome.

Silvery hair: Silvery decoloration of hair as a marker of Chediak-Higashi, Griscelli, and Elejande syndromes.

Spunglass hair: Rough dry aspect of hair found in uncombable hair syndrome.

Straight hair nevus: Localized straight hair on curly hair pattern.

Trichobezoar: Compact mass of hair on the stomach resulting from eating hair.

Trichodaganomania: Compulsive habit of biting one's own hair.

Trichodinia: Hair or scalp pain experienced by some patients.

Trichomalacia: Deformed and swollen hair caused by repeated trauma usually found in trichotillomania.

Trichonodosis: Single or complex knots of hair usually provoked by compulsive manual handling.

Trichophagia: Compulsive hair eating; usually associated with trichotillomania.

Trichoptilosis: Acquired distal splitting of hair shafts usually associated with distal trichorrhexis nodosa in long hair styles.

Trichorrhexis invaginata: Introduction of a distal hair shaft into a proximal hair shaft as in a bowel invagination; pathognomonic of Netherton syndrome.

Trichorrhexis nodosa: Nodes of hair fracture, expose the cortex, and cause brush-like ends on fibers. Acquired trichorrhexis nodosa is common. Familial cases of proximal trichorrhexis nodosa and acquired distal dystrophic forms have been described.

Trichorrhizophagia: Habit of eating the roots of plucked hairs.

Trichoschisis: Sharp, transverse fracture characteristic of trichothiodystrophy.

Trichosclasis: Irregular oblique hair fracture.

Trichoteiromania: Perpetual rubbing of the scalp causing fracturing of hair shafts.

Trichotemnomania: Hair loss caused by cutting or shaving.

Trichothiodystrophy: Complex syndrome characterized by sulfur-deficient hair that shows a zebra-like aspect under polarized light microscopy and trichoschisis; usually associated with ichthyosis.

Trichotillomania: Compulsive disorder characterized by self-extraction of hair.

Tufted folliculitis: Chronic scalp inflammation in which several follicles exit the skin through a single opening.

Whisker hair: Acquired localized form of curly hair seen in temporal areas.

Woolly hair: Thin, curly hair, flat in transverse section that simulates Negroid hair but is thinner than normal; several forms recognized include diffuse and localized (woolly hair nevus).

Yellow dots: Protrusions of sebaceous glands of the empty follicles onto the skin surface; they appear as yellow dots seen in patches of alopecia areata.

Appendix: Silvery Hair Syndromes

Silvery hairs are cutaneous markers of Chediak-Higashi, Elejalde, and Griscelli syndromes that are congenital recessive trait conditions of childhood onset with neurological involvement [1]. These conditions are associated with mutations of various genes that encode several proteins involved in the intracellular processing and movement of melanosomes. They are characterized by the silvery aspect of the hair shaft (Figure A.1) and partial albinism and can be differentiated easily by the distribution of hair melanin granules (Figures A.2a and b) and immunity involvement (Table A.1) [2–4]. Sporadic transient silvery hair associated with congenital hydrops fetalis and hypoproteinemia has been reported [5]. Table A.1 shows the differential diagnosis of these conditions.

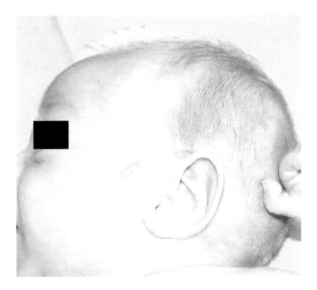

FIGURE A.1 Characteristic aspect of silvery hair in patient. (From Galve J, Martín-Santiago A, Clavero C et al. Spontaneous repigmentation of silvery hair in an infant with congenital hydrops fetalis and hypoproteinemia. Accepted by *Cutis*, 2015.

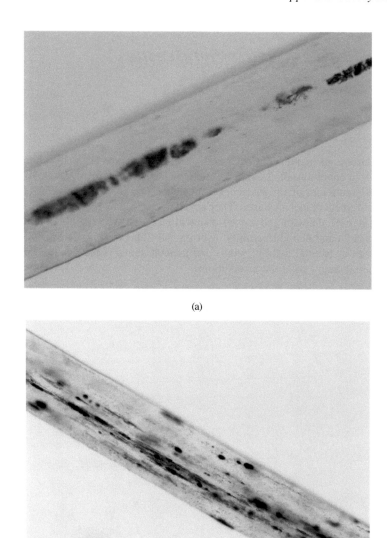

(a)

(b)

FIGURE A.2   Peculiar distribution of pigment on hair shaft in (a) Chediak-Higashi syndrome and (b) Elejalde or Griscelli syndrome.

TABLE A.1

Differential Diagnosis of Silvery Hair Conditions

	Syndrome		
Symptom	**Griscelli**	**Chediak-Higashi**	**Elejalde**
Leukocytic granules	Present	Not present	Not present
Recurrent infection	Frequent	Rare	Frequent
Hair melanin	Small regular granules	Large and small irregular granules	Large and small irregular granules
Skin melanin	Large granules with pigmentation of basal layer	Irregular-size granules and giant melanosomes	Irregular distribution
Immunity	Decrease of chemotaxis	Not involved	Immediate and delayed

REFERENCES

1. Sahana M, Sacchidanand S, Hiremagalore R et al. Silvery grey hair: clue to diagnosing immunodeficiency. *J Trichology* 4: 83–85, 2012.
2. Raghuveer C, Murthy SC, Mithuna MN et al. Silvery hair with speckled dyspigmentation: Chediak-Higashi syndrome in three Indian siblings. *J Trichology* 7: 133–135, 2015.
3. Nouriel A, Zisquit J, Helfand AM et al. Griscelli syndrome type 3: two new cases and review of the literature. *Pediatr Dermatol* 32: 245–248, 2015.
4. Cahali JB, Fernandez SA, Oliveira ZN et al. Elejalde syndrome: report of a case and review of the literature. *Pediatr Dermatol* 21: 479–482, 2004.
5. Galve J, Martín-Santiago A, Clavero C et al. Spontaneous repigmentation of silvery hair in an infant with congenital hydrops fetalis and hypoproteinemia. Accepted by *Cutis*, 2015.

Index

T - #0920 - 101024 - C110 - 254/178/5 - PB - 9781498707770 - Gloss Lamination